2nd edition

Pass the
MRCPsych

(Parts I and II)

Provided as a service to medicine by
Eli Lilly and Company Limited

Commissioning Editor: Michael Parkinson
Project Manager: Fiona Conn
Design: Typearea (Falkirk)

2nd edition

Pass the MRCPsych
(Parts I and II)

All the techniques you need

Christopher Williams
Peter Trigwell
David Yeomans

W.B. SAUNDERS

Edinburgh • London • New york • Philadelphia • Sydney • Toronto 2000

W.B. SAUNDERS
An imprint of Elsevier Science Limited

First edition 1995
Second edition first published 2000
  Reprinted 2002

ISBN 0702025429

British Library Cataloguing in Publication Data
A catalogue record for this book is available from the British Library

Library of Congress Cataloging in Publication Data
A catalog record for this book is available from the Library of Congress

Note
Medical knowledge is constantly changing. As new information becomes available, changes in treatment, procedures, equipment and the use of drugs become necessary. The authors and the publishers have taken care to ensure that the information given in this text is accurate and up to date. However, readers are strongly advised to confirm that the information, especially with regard to drug usage, complies with the latest legislation and standards of practice.

The
publisher's
policy is to use
**paper manufactured
from sustainable forests**

Printed in China by RDC Group Limited

Contents

Contributors

Dr Christopher Williams
Senior Lecturer/Honorary Consultant in Psychiatry,
University of Glasgow, Academic Centre,
Gartnavel Royal Hospital, Glasgow G12 0XH, UK

Dr Peter Trigwell
Consultant in Liaison Psychiatry, Leeds General Infirmary,
Great George Street, Leeds LS1 3EX, UK

Dr David Yeomans
Consultant Psychiatrist, Overthorpe House, 226 Otley Road,
Leeds LS16 5AB, UK

Dr Kevin Appleton
Child and Adolescent Psychiatrist, Marinoto West,
Waitakere Hospital, Auckland, New Zealand

Dr David Protheroe
Consultant Psychiatrist, Department of Psychiatry, The Northern Hospital,
185 Cooper Street, Epping 3076, Australia

Dr Keith Brownlee
Consultant Paediatrician, St James's University Hospital, Beckett Street,
Leeds LS9 7TF, UK

Dr Catherine Brown
Specialist Registrar in Child and Adolescent Psychiatry, Child and Adolescent
Services, Fieldhead House, 228 St Martin's Avenue, Fieldhead Business Centre,
Listerhills, Bradford BD7 1LG, UK

Foreword

Even more people now wish to pass the MRCPsych examination than when the first edition of this book was published. Readers will find this edition both readable and accessible and that it helps them to make the most of the professional knowledge and clinical skills that they already have. It is not intended, primarily, to teach facts but to help candidates present what they know with precision and lucidity. It has been developed from a highly successful course for MRCPsych candidates – highly successful in both the numbers clamouring to attend the course, and in an excellent pass rate.

A relatively difficult examination is not only a rite of passage for joining the ranks of psychiatrists, it is also a test of motivation and a guarantee to future patients that the successful candidate has acquired the necessary knowledge and skills. This book encourages clarity of thought, marshalling of the factual information that the trainee psychiatrist already has, and expression of facts and opinions in terms that are comprehensible to candidate and examiner alike. For this reason it does not only contribute to passing the examination, but also assists in the transition from a junior doctor studying psychiatry, to an able and therapeutically effective trained psychiatrist. I would, therefore, commend *Pass the MRCPsych*, 2nd edition, not only to candidates for the examination but also to their teachers, clinical tutors and educational supervisors.

Professor A C P Sims, MA MD FRCP (London & Edinburgh) FCPS (Pakistan)
Division of Psychiatry and Behavioural Sciences in Relation to Medicine,
Clinical Sciences Building, St James's University Hospital, Leeds LS9 7TF, UK

Introduction

Clinical competence and passing the Membership Examinations for the Royal College of Psychiatrists are the most visible criteria by which trainees progress up the career ladder in psychiatry. Taking the examinations is costly in both financial and personal terms. To pass requires very significant work and commitment.

In writing this second edition, we have updated and revised the contents of the book. We are pleased that the first edition was well received, and that we have this opportunity to respond to recent changes in the examination structure. Two completely new chapters on the subject of the 'Critical Review Paper' introduced in Spring 1999 have been added. We have also altered and re-edited all remaining chapters based on feedback and comments from the past four years of the Leeds Examination Techniques Course.

In common with the first edition, this book is not a 'crammer' book of key facts for the examination. You will find that very few factual pieces of information are presented. Instead, it will help you to present the information that you have learned elsewhere (whether from formal revision, everyday psychiatric practice or other sources) in a professional and structured way. Even very good clinicians with a strong factual knowledge fail the examinations because of poor technique. This book will help you use your knowledge and experience effectively to enable you to pass.

We hope that you will find our book helpful. In producing any book such as this, many other people are always involved. We wish to acknowledge the help and support of the various tutors, lecturers and examiners who have contributed to the development of the Leeds Examination Techniques Course and the associated books.

Finally, but most importantly, we wish to thank Alison, Amanda and Frances for their support and understanding during the writing of this book.

Chris Williams, Peter Trigwell, David Yeomans
March 2000

Important practical and preparation issues

David Yeomans and Peter Trigwell

Structure of the MRCPsych Parts I and II

Part I

To apply, candidates must have completed 12 months of full-time (or equivalent part-time) approved training. Full details of how to apply are to be found in the College *General Information and Regulations for the MRCPsych Examinations.*

The Part I exam currently comprises a multiple choice question (MCQ) paper and a clinical examination.

Part I MCQ Paper

50-question MCQ paper to be answered in 90 minutes. Each question has five stems. The topics covered are:

- Psychology: basic psychology, social psychology, neuropsychology, psychological assessment
- Human development
- Psychopathology
- Psychopharmacology: general principles
- Pharmacokinetics
- Pharmacodynamics
- Adverse drug reactions.

NB At the time of writing neuroanatomy, neuropathology, neurophysiology and neurochemistry are **not** examined in the Part I exam. However, this paper is liable to change incrementally over the next few years.

This paper is marked using **neutral marking**, so that a mark is gained for every correct response you make. Any incorrect response or question that is left blank scores zero points.

Part I Clinical Examination

This is outlined in detail in Chapters 7 and 8. You will have an hour with the patient and then be examined on the case for 30 minutes. The Part I clinical includes the assessment of patients, but excludes clinical management.

The clinical examination will be based on a case from one of the following, or a combination of these:

- General adult psychiatry
- Hospital liaison psychiatry
- Old age psychiatry
- Substance misuse.

To be successful, the candidate must pass the Clinical Examination and achieve a standard in the MCQ paper that is acceptable to the College. Candidates are allowed a maximum of between two and four attempts at the MRCPsych Part I examination (depending on the duration of the previous approved psychiatric training). For more details see *General Information and Regulations for the MRCPsych Examinations*, which will be sent to you when you apply to sit the exams. The College revises the Examination procedure at intervals; *it is essential for each candidate to get the most up to date guidelines.*

Part II

To apply, candidates must have passed or be exempted from the MRCPsych Part I and have completed 30 months full-time (or equivalent part-time) approved training. Full details of how to apply are to be found in the College *General Information and Regulations for the MRCPsych Examinations.*

The Part II exam currently comprises several written papers and two clinical examinations.

Part II Written Papers
- 50-question MCQ paper (90 minutes) on clinical topics (neutral marking).
- 50-question MCQ paper (90 minutes) on sciences basic to psychiatry (neutral marking).
- Critical review paper (CRP) to assess the candidate's critical appraisal skills (45 minutes).
- Essay paper (90 minutes total). Two questions must be answered: one question from two on general psychiatry and one question from two on the psychiatric specialties (child and adolescent psychiatry, forensic psychiatry, mental handicap, psychiatry of old age and psychotherapy).

Part II Clinical Examination
This is made up of two sections: the 'long case' **individual patient assessment** (one hour with the patient and 30 minutes with the examiners) and the **patient management problems** (PMPs, lasting 30 minutes).

To be successful, candidates must pass the Clinical Examination and achieve a standard in the other sections which is acceptable to the College.

Candidates are allowed a maximum of five attempts at the MRCPsych Part II examination. For more details see *General Information and Regulations for the MRCPsych Examinations* which will be sent to you when you apply to sit the exams. The College revises the Examination procedure at intervals; *it is essential for each candidate to get the most up to date guidelines.*

There are significant changes proposed to both parts of the exam and it cannot be over-emphasised how important it is to obtain the up to date College syllabus in order to find out what areas of knowledge you will be expected to have. Surveys have shown that it is surprisingly rare for people to send off for this syllabus and read it once it has arrived.

Applying to sit the exam

Before taking the exam you will need to find two 'sponsors'. One must be your clinical tutor and the other a consultant who you have worked with for at least four months during the year prior to the date of application. The deadline for getting your application in is surprisingly early; you need to request the forms from the College several months in advance.

Preparation

Once you have decided when to take the exam you will need to work out a timetable for your revision. This can help you to identify what work needs to be covered. It will also help to keep you on target for the exam if you stick to your timetable. Most people assign a period of 2–3 months for revision for Part I, and 3–6 months for Part II. It is best to work consistently, e.g. two hours a night, but be flexible to allow for relaxation, on-call commitments, and other occasions. It can be helpful to decide upon a day each week when you will definitely **not** revise. Regular breaks help to maintain commitment the rest of the time.

It may help to structure your revision timetable by following the contents of one of the major textbooks. You will also need a checklist of the subject areas in the syllabus to ensure that you cover everything required.

Practice

An analysis of your learning style, as described in the next chapter, will shape the way you prepare for the exams. Practice is essential in preparing for each component of the exam. It is important to test yourself regularly throughout the revision period in order to get feedback on your performance. For Part I you will need to practise multiple choice questions (MCQs) and clinical assessment and presentation. For Part II you will also need to practise writing structured essays, critical appraisal of literature (CRP) and reasoned solutions to patient management problems (PMPs). All these features should be built into your revision timetable as well as your learning of basic information.

Familiarity with the actual exam can only be gained through practice. Be assertive in your pursuit of exam practice. Ask senior colleagues to listen to your presentations and give feedback. Each person you ask will have a slightly different opinion on what is good and bad about your efforts. Practice will help you to build up confidence in your abilities before you enter the examination room.

Mental health

Examinations cause stress over an extended period. It is worthwhile considering how the process is affecting you. Do you need a break? What about a holiday or a night out? If you do suffer from exam nerves it pays to practise relaxation beforehand. Although some people have been known to find anxiolytics helpful, medication should generally be avoided. Last minute revision is sometimes more of an anxiolytic than an aid to memory. Do it if you wish to, but a day of rest before the exams can also be helpful.

Getting ready for the exam

Get study leave arranged well in advance. Consider a revision course prior to the exam. It is often helpful to take a week off work just before the exam to do final preparations. Do not be persuaded to cover for an absent colleague at the last moment; you have spent too much time, effort and money to let personnel issues get in the way.

Find a decent place to stay before the exam. Do not skimp on last minute comforts, especially if you can claim expenses. Give yourself plenty of time to travel. It is better to arrive two hours early than two minutes late.

With good preparation you can feel confident that the exam is not going to bring up too many surprises and that you can comfortably cope with any that do arise. When doing the exam, although you will feel some anxiety, good preparation should prevent you being thrown off balance by a difficult question, or at least enable you to function on 'auto-pilot' until you regain your equilibrium. If you follow the advice in this book, you will have pre-prepared answers and answering techniques for difficult questions. You will know how to impress examiners by your presentation technique. You will know the ins and outs of the exam structure and how it is marked. You will know what is expected of you. All this will help reduce your anxiety and improve your exam performance.

After the exam

Certain parts of the exam, such as the 'basic sciences' MCQ paper in Part II, leave many candidates feeling that they have probably failed (although many have passed). These feelings may continue for some time. Try to avoid too many post-mortems. Try to avoid talking in detail about how the exam has gone to others, particularly during the breaks between the different written and clinical exams in Part II. Going over your answers again and again in your mind analysing possible mistakes is rarely helpful.

You have to wait a while for the results. A holiday away immediately after the exams may be a good idea. If you pass, well done! If not, then **try again** as many members of the Royal College have had to do before. Use the feedback from examiners and keep working on exam techniques. (See Chapter 10: '*If at first you don't succeed . . . '*.)

Key points
- Obtain and read the exam regulations and information for candidates.
- Understand how they apply to you.
- When you have decided to take the exam, send off for the application forms early.
- Submit completed forms, with the appropriate fee, in good time.
- Formulate a comprehensive revision timetable,

---

including time off for recreation, etc.
- Examination technique can help you communicate what you know to your best ability. Think carefully about this aspect of the exam.
- Practise.

REFERENCES

It is important to obtain and read the following Royal College publications:

1. *Handbook for Inceptors and Trainees in Psychiatry,*
   Royal College of Psychiatrists

2. *General Information and Regulations for the MRCPsych Examinations,*
   Royal College of Psychiatrists

3. *Past Papers in Psychiatry,*
   Royal College of Psychiatrists.

These can be obtained from the Royal College of Psychiatrists, 17 Belgrave Square, London SW1X 8PG, UK. Tel: (020) 7235 2351.

Learning styles and revision strategies

Peter Trigwell and David Yeomans

It is often believed that success in medical examinations simply depends upon the regurgitation of facts. This is not true. It is possible to know the facts of a subject very well and still fail the examination. You can improve your exam performance with good technique. Technique refers to your style of learning and preparing, and then of presenting what you know to best effect.

Consider the nature of your personal learning style. Different people have different preferred learning styles.[1] Some may have a

---

Preferred learning styles

Serialistic learning style:
- Follow a step by step linear progression from one item of information to another
- Focus on only one aspect of the problem at one time
- Focus on facts and logic
- Tend to prefer a linear delivery of material (e.g. by attending a lecture or reading a textbook).

Global/holistic learning style:
- Readiness to think divergently
- Examine several aspects of the current problem
- Formulate more complex hypotheses
- Make use of wider previous experience and link this to the new area
- Tend to prefer use of analogies and links to prior experience.

---

serialistic approach and others a more global/holistic approach to learning. These different styles appear to be stable over time and are summarised in the box on page 9.

The following is a list of questions about learning style. Work through it point by point; it is designed to encourage you to think about how you learn.

- Do you revise in a **suitable environment**? (– quiet, warm enough, well lit, minimum of disturbance). How can you **improve** the environment?
- Do you **structure your learning**? (– according to the Royal College syllabus). See *Handbook for Inceptors and Trainees.*[2]
- Do you know what **sources of information** you are most comfortable with? This is likely to relate to your basic learning style.
- **How much information** can you take in at one go? There is no point staring at a book when your concentration seems to have gone. Taking a break will also allow consolidation of what you have learned.
- **How much repetition** do you need? Does it help to read several accounts from differing books, perhaps followed by a re-read of your own notes to fix those facts in your memory? Alternatively, are you the type of person who prefers to learn just one or two books really well?
- Do you **set goals**? (– learn the components of the cranial nerves today and test yourself tomorrow).
- Do you **achieve these goals**?
- Do you **review your progress**? (– plan and write out a **clear revision timetable**, and try to stick to it so that you do not run out of time).
- Can you **prioritise**? (– learn the common things before the esoteric).
- Do you **keep the exam in mind while learning**? (– in order to memorise information in the style appropriate to the exam).
- Do you **use your daily work to help you learn**? (– reflecting on your differential diagnoses, formulations, and management plans, and presenting cases under exam conditions).

- Are you **adequately motivated**? (– try to make this positive, e.g. career progression or self satisfaction, rather than negative, e.g. because it is 'expected' by others).
- Do you **use others to help you learn**? Do you work best by yourself, or as part of a group? Many find that a combination of approaches is most effective. Consider meeting once weekly for several hours with other colleagues who are doing the exam. **Study groups** like this may provide support as well as assisting with your revision.

Condensing information

There is a large amount of information to learn, particularly for Part II, and certainly too much to review it all in the few days leading up to the exam. A number of techniques are available to aid rapid review of key information.

Reducing the quantity of information in books/written materials
- Emphasise key areas of text (highlighters, underline etc.).
- Cross irrelevant or unclear materials out.
- Add new materials to margins.

Make notes
- Relatively long (such as writing out many sheets of A4) or short notes (e.g. key words/bullet points) may be used.
- These can be used to either replace or supplement books.

Other aids to remembering
- Making lists of key information can help you to generate and impose a structure on what you learn.
- Consider reinforcing your learning by using MCQs or writing an essay to test your learning.

You may find that your ability to remember clinical topics/materials is enhanced by:
- Learning cases/management based around a clinical structure (PC/ HPC, etc.)

- Imagining or writing down details of a 'typical' case that summarises all the important principles of assessment or management
- Remembering a specific patient who encompasses a typical or atypical presentation, assessment or clinical management plan.

Another possible approach is the use of Mind Maps® to summarise and structure your learning (see the Appendix).

Appropriate sources of information

Part I

Many people have found it possible to pass the Part I examination using a group of small books such as those listed below. These books are suggestions only, but reflect the sort of level of knowledge and understanding which are required for this exam.

Suitable textbooks/Part I exam

- *Examination Notes in Psychiatry* (Buckley, Bird and Harrison)[3] or another 'core book'.
- *Introduction to Psychotherapy* (Brown and Pedder).[4]
- *Examination Notes for the MRCPsych Part I* (Puri and Sklar)[5] – for neurosciences, etc.
- *Symptoms in the Mind* (Sims)[6] – for psychopathology.
- *ICD 10* (World Health Organization).[7]

It is also worthwhile reading relevant sections of the *British National Formulary* (BNF). This contains an up to date summary of current prescribing practice.

Part II

For Part II you may need to decide early on whether you prefer to comprehensively learn a large, up to date text (e.g. *Companion to Psychiatric Studies*[8]) supplemented by some journal papers, or use a mixture of smaller books and rather more journal papers. Do not forget to concentrate on the main areas; these are often overlooked as people become bogged down in the fine detail of more obscure topics. Learn psychology and sociology **early**. These are key areas, particularly for the 'basic sciences' MCQ paper, and they take quite some time to revise. You should try and avoid the (common) situation where candidates try to learn these subjects from scratch with only a month or so to go.

Key points

- Passing the exam requires a clear revision strategy.
- Exam techniques can be vital.
- Think about the way you learn – is it as effective as it could be?
- Revise with the exam in mind.
- Use your daily work to help you learn.
- Practice is essential.

REFERENCES

1. Flett A (1996) Student personality and approaches to learning. *Teaching and Learning Occasional Paper No 1*. Leicester University: Leicester.

2. *Handbook for Inceptors and Trainees*. This is available from: The Royal College of Psychiatrists, 17 Belgrave Square, London SW1X 8PG, UK. Tel: (020) 7235 2351.

3. Buckley P, Bird J, Harrison G (1985) *Examination Notes in Psychiatry*, Third Edition. Butterworth Heinemann: Oxford.

4. Brown D, Pedder J (1989) *Introduction to Psychotherapy*. Routledge: London.

5. Puri B, Sklar J (1989) *Examination Notes for the MRCPsych Part I*. Butterworths: London.

6. Sims A (1995) *Symptoms in the Mind. An Introduction to Descriptive Psychopathology*, Second Edition. WB Saunders: London.

7. World Health Organization (1992) *The ICD10 Classification of Mental and Behavioural Disorders*. WHO: Geneva.

8. Johnstone E, Freeman CPL, Zealley AK (1998) *Companion to Psychiatric Studies*, Sixth Edition. Churchill Livingstone: Edinburgh.

MCQ technique

Christopher Williams, David Protheroe and Keith Brownlee

The MCQ paper is the most structured of the MRCPsych exams. It aims to test the candidate's factual knowledge and knowledge of the finer detail of the subject quickly and reliably. Trainee doctors can fail the MRCPsych Part I or II exam as a result of poor MCQ technique. This chapter suggests ways of planning your learning with the MCQ exam in mind and also describes methods to improve your MCQ technique so that you are able to use your knowledge more effectively.

Make sure that you understand the mark scheme. The exam is marked using a **neutral marking scheme**. This allocates marks accordingly:

Response	Score
Correct answer	+1
Blank response	0
Incorrect answer	0

What should I learn?

Obtain and read the Royal College guidelines about the content of the exam.

Part I MCQ contents
Know how the exam is structured. At the time of writing, candidates are required to answer 50 questions in 90 minutes:

- Psychology: basic psychology, social psychology, neuropsychology, psychological assessment

- Human development
- Psychopathology
- Psychopharmacology: general principles, pharmacokinetics, pharmacodynamics, adverse drug reactions.

NB At the time of writing neuroanatomy, neuropathology, neurophysiology and neurochemistry are **not** examined in the Part I exam.

Part II MCQ contents

- **Basic sciences**: 50 questions in 90 minutes.
- **Clinical**: 50 questions in 90 minutes. Be prepared for it: there may be a substantial number of questions on various sub-specialties.

The content of the Part II paper is very broad. Obtain the document *The Basic Sciences and Clinical Curricula for the MRCPsych Examinations* from the Royal College Examinations Department.

Preparing for the MCQ exam

- Produce a clear revision timetable in order to cover each area of the exam adequately. You will need to start your revision **well before** the exam if you are going to cover all the subject areas.
- It is often useful to go on a **revision course** at the very beginning of your revision. There are several advantages to this. It can help you get your revision going, boost your motivation and highlight areas of weakness on which to focus your learning. It allows you to realise the depth of knowledge that you must aim for and the amount of time you need to set aside for your revision.

Using MCQs to help you revise

Although there is no substitute for a thorough understanding of the subject matter, MCQs can be useful to help you revise and learn.

- At the beginning of your preparation for the exam it is useful to spend some time **writing** multiple choice questions. For example, after completing a chapter of a book, try to write a few MCQ questions on the subject you have just learned. This helps to **re-inforce** and test your knowledge and will help **highlight** the kind of information which is amenable to MCQs. The questions are also useful for later revision.

- As you read through your textbooks, mark facts which are MCQ-able with a **highlighter pen**. The number of black and white or true/false facts are remarkably limited. This will help you focus your learning.
- Remember that the information needed to answer MCQs is quite different from that needed to 'manage a patient'.

Using MCQs to help you learn

A large variety of MCQ books are available. Some of these are better (and more accurate) than others. Some books contain whole papers of mixed questions; others consist of questions organised by topic. Both of these formats are very helpful, but should be used in different ways.

- Make your revision more interesting by using MCQs. Some people find that when they continually revise a set of notes over a period of weeks they cease to take any new information in. One way of preventing this is to practise MCQs on each topic shortly after you have revised it.
- Remember that MCQ books and papers can help identify the sort of information which is asked in MCQ exams. **Improve your factual knowledge base** by reading and testing yourself with as many MCQs as you can. If you find you do badly in a particular subject or topic, target your reading towards these areas. You can then re-read the topic looking for the answers to the questions that you got wrong. This helps highlight particular areas of a subject as important, and allows you to add important details to your notes.
- Do not try to remember hundreds of dislocated facts. Instead try to **integrate** information you learn with your existing knowledge so that you **understand the principles** involved. **Summary notes** may help you do this. Of most value are those books which **explain** the answers so that you add to your knowledge.

Subject spotting

Exam courses often emphasise subject spotting. By analysing previous papers and reporting the apparent frequency of different subjects, it is suggested that it is possible to target revision at specific exam-orientated subjects. This is generally of limited value as the content of different exams varies significantly. It is clear, however, that there are certain core subject areas that you must know and understand well. For example, it can be very tempting for candidates approaching the exam to 'put off' revising psychology, sociology, human development and statistics. Try to avoid making the mistake of leaving these topics until just before the exam. These areas are large and need to be learned well. **It is not possible to revise them in only one or two days**.

Trust your 'feeling of knowing'

In the MCQ, one mark will be awarded for each correct answer and zero marks for an incorrect response. In theory, if you haven't a clue about the answer, a complete guess should have an equal chance of being correct or incorrect thus resulting in an average of 50 marks. In practice, however, some people seem to be naturally better at answering MCQ questions than others and will score highly because of their ability to make a **confident calculated guess**. One area which has been researched is the 'feeling of knowing' that candidates experience when they read certain questions. When you do an MCQ paper, you will find that you:

- **Know** the answer with a high degree of certainty
- Definitely know that you **don't know** the answer
- Have a '**feeling of knowing**' that the answer is correct, but are not quite sure.

In a neutrally marked paper you must answer all the questions; **don't leave any blank**.

> **Please note**: If you are someone who has a high level of confidence in your answers, and yet more often than not gets them wrong, this shows that you need to improve your factual knowledge.

Can you say 'no'?

Overall you should be confident about your 'true' answers; after all you are answering it as 'true' because you have seen or heard it somewhere before. It is much more difficult to be confident about your 'false' answers – the fact that you think that 'A is not a feature of B' may simply reflect that you do not know much about the subject! **Candidates are less likely to answer a question if the correct answer is 'false' than if it is 'true'.** Therefore being able to correctly answer the 'false' questions can give you the edge over other candidates, and be a very valuable source of extra marks.

The confidence test

Complete several MCQ papers using your normal answering style. Repeat the papers after changing your strategy by answering more questions which you feel are wrong as false. Compare your marks with your usual answering style. **Do you gain or lose marks using this technique?** If you are consistently gaining marks, you should actively consider altering your threshold of response.

In addition, consider carrying out a more detailed analysis on your answers on several papers. Try to identify if there are **areas of knowledge** in which you have a particularly low level or high level of confidence (e.g. you may have a greater confidence in psychopathology than in drug treatments, etc.).

MCQ technique

Timing and practical issues

Check the up to date College examination instructions and regulations to find out how many questions you have to complete and what time is allocated. The structure and content of the exam may change. At the time of writing, the MCQ papers in both Part I and II of the exam consist of 50 questions to be completed in 90 minutes. This means that there are 1.8 minutes per question available.

- **Read the whole question very carefully** and break it down into individual facts. Mark each of these facts as true or false. Read each stem and item as a single sentence.
- Be particularly careful with questions on topics about which you are confident. Your elation may lead you to misread the question and lose marks where you should have gained them.
- Have you understood the question? Beware of double negatives – one in the question and one in the stem.
- Make sure you put each answer **straight away** onto the **right line** of the marking sheet. Review this every few questions. It is easy to get your answers out of order. This will cause panic and could cost you the exam.
- Ruthlessly **skip** those questions where you really don't know the answer and come back to them later. You may find that other questions trigger your memory, and the answer will come back to you as the exam continues. If you still have no idea make a guess response. By the law of averages, a complete guess will score you 50% of the available marks. **Do not leave questions blank at the end of the exam**.
- Review your progress and maintain momentum. You should be aiming to finish every 10 questions in approximately 15 minutes. This allows you time at the end to review your answers.
- Regularly (say every 10 questions, **check that you have transcribed the answers onto the correct line on the answer sheet**.
- Consider whether to stay in or leave the room when you have completed the paper. Many people benefit by staying and going through the paper one more time. **Again, make sure you have made an answer to every question**.

Don't be too clever

- Do not automatically assume that the examiners are trying to trick you. Avoid agonising over possible hidden meanings, as this is more likely to hinder rather than help your decisions.
- In MCQs, the 'correct' answer to a question is the **generally accepted version of the truth**. If you have some special know-

ledge of a topic that is at variance with the most prevalent view point – swallow your pride and save it for the essay paper!

MCQ example strategies

The following facts about our solar system are true:
a) It takes 365 days for the Earth to orbit the Sun
b) The same side of the Moon is always visible from the Earth
c) The moon circles the Earth every 28 days
d) Gravity is related to the speed of rotation of a planet
e) Only planets with an iron core have a magnetic field.

- The answer to stem **a)** is true. However, the very knowledgeable candidate may be aware that the Earth takes 365.27 days to circulate the Sun; this candidate may therefore answer false. 365 is **near enough right** and should be marked as true.

- The same side of the Moon is always visible from Earth, therefore stem **b)** is true. However, there is a phenomenon called libration, as a consequence of which 59% of the Moon's surface is visible, but at different times. If a candidate is aware of this they may then answer this question incorrectly as false. This is reading too much into the question.

- The answer to stem **c)** is true. However, as with stem **a)**, the very knowledgeable candidate may be aware that the Moon takes 27.3 days to circulate the Earth; they may then answer this as false. This is being too precise: 28 days is near enough to the correct answer to be marked true.

- The answer to stem **d)** is false. Gravity is related to the mass of an object. This is a question you can only answer if you have specific knowledge about this fact.

- **Dichotomous words** such as 'only' and 'always' and 'never' often indicate that the answer is false. It is very rare for a finding to **only** occur in one single situation. The answer to stem **e)** is therefore likely to be (and in fact is) false. This is not foolproof however – see stem **b)**.

The numbers game

- There is no set pass mark. A candidate's performance is compared to all other candidates taking the exam on that occasion.
- If you are finding the paper horrendously difficult it is likely that others are too. **Do not give up**. Carry on and try to finish. Do not leave the exam hall in despair. You can still pass.
- **Don't waste time counting your answers**; you really don't know how many you have correct. Answer every question to the best of your ability.

Be aware of the techniques examiners use in writing questions

It is surprisingly difficult to write good MCQs. Understanding some of the techniques used will help you to avoid some of the possible pitfalls. It is useful to think about questions from the perspective of the person writing them. They will wish to have a spread of true and false responses, of varying degrees of difficulty. Ideally the questions will be able to discriminate between those who know a subject well and those whose knowledge is superficial.

It is relatively easy to formulate 'true' questions. Read a chapter in a textbook and see how easy it is to pick out five facts that are true. The question can be made more difficult either by choosing obscure facts or by expressing the question in a form that is unlikely to have been read in a textbook, but can be worked out if the subject is known well. It is possible that you will sometimes know the answer to a question but not realise it. This is because the question has been **phrased in an unexpected way** or because it occurs in an unexpected place.

It is much more difficult for the examiners to write good 'false' questions. They may be created by using **popular misconceptions** or by using the **opposite** of the truth. The examiners will write the question by '*switching*' information that is found in sources such as textbooks.

Recognising the 'switch'

The following can be switched:

1. Nouns (or diseases)
2. Adjectives
3. Negative to positive, or vice versa.

Example of 'switching' in MCQs

The following statements about the planets are true:
a) Jupiter has a great dark spot
b) The hottest planet is Mercury.

- The answer to stem **a)** is false. If the candidate remembers that Jupiter has a spot he may well answer this as true; unfortunately for him Jupiter has a **red** spot, Neptune has a dark spot. This stem has been created by **switching words** or by **mixing known facts**.
- The answer to stem **b)** is false. If the candidate knows that Mercury is the nearest planet to the sun, she may answer this question as true. Venus, the second nearest planet to the sun is, however, the hottest as Venus possesses an atmosphere and, unlike Mercury, is affected by the greenhouse effect. This question has been created by **switching key words**.

The wording of the question

It is important to look at questions from two perspectives: factual knowledge and logic. However, good MCQs are difficult to write and many questions contain some clues within the structure of the question. Use your common sense.

Three particularly common stems are:

1. A '**characteristic feature**' means that it is of diagnostic significance. Its absence might make one doubt the diagnosis. If it is truly characteristic then you are likely to be aware of it
2. A '**typical feature**' is one that you would expect to be present. It is similar to 'characteristic'

3. A '**recognised feature**' is one that, although it may not charac-
terise a disease, has been reported. Marking this as false implies
an in-depth knowledge of the subject, unless it can be recognised
as a switch.

Other terminology

- ' . . . **is a pathognomonic feature**' means it occurs only in that
  condition. If you do not know the answer then it is likely to be
  false. There are few pathognomonic features and you are likely
  to know them.
- ' . . . **is associated with**' means that it is a feature which is well
  recognised but not common. The same applies to a '. . . **is a
  recognised feature of**'.
- Categorical answers such as '**Never, always, only, invariably**'
  should usually be answered as **false**, unless you are sure that
  they are true. Such absolute statements are rarely correct.

Use your sense of logic

The following techniques may help you clarify your thinking about
an answer:

1. Look for terminology that is likely to make a question true or false
2. Beware of double negatives
3. Reversing the question (e.g. 'X **may not** occur in Y') can help
   clarify your thinking. Try this with some questions in any MCQ
   book to illustrate how helpful this technique is
4. Look for items which are **contradictory** or the same.
   Contradictory items should not be included within one question
   as they will be immediately obvious. However, they may be
   included in different questions, and this can offer you additional
   clues.

It is important to remember that virtually none of the current MCQ
books on the market seems to be as difficult as the Part II MCQ
papers. If you feel that you have done badly on any one paper, **don't
worry!** Particularly on the Part II basic sciences paper, it is normal to
think you have done badly. Remember that your overall MCQ mark
compares your score with everyone else's, and that if you have

found that the paper has been very hard, it is likely that everyone else will have as well.

Key points

- Make sure you know the structure of the exam.
- Start your revision early.
- Practise using a variety of MCQ books and use MCQs to help you revise.
- Initially concentrate on a solid understanding of the subject matter.
- Start concentrating on MCQ-able facts at least 6–8 weeks before the exam.
- Work to perfect your technique.
- Read the questions very carefully.
- Don't panic: exam papers are often very difficult.
- Read the questions carefully, looking for clues in the wording.
- Keep checking your answers are in the correct place on the answer sheet.
- Maintain momentum.
- Using these techniques may help you gain some further marks, but there is no substitute for developing broad-based knowledge.

The critical review paper

David Yeomans

Introduction

The critical review paper (CRP) was introduced in Spring 1999. It is a 90-minute written paper. The paper is divided into two parts, one with 70% and the other with 30% of the marks. Each part contains an abridged account of a research project and related questions. The questions examine your knowledge of research methods. You will be asked to critically appraise the studies presented.

Few exam candidates have become experienced researchers by the time they sit this paper. Their knowledge of critical appraisal is therefore theoretical rather than experiential. Fortunately there are many sources of basic advice on statistics and critical appraisal, and journal clubs should provide a forum in which trainees can develop their skills and confidence in this area.

This chapter aims to help familiarise readers with the aims and requirements of the CRP, which have been clearly set out by the Royal College of Psychiatrists in their *MRCPsych Part II Guidance Notes*,[1] *The Critical Review Paper Information Pack*[2] and *The Basic Sciences and Clinical Curricula*.[3]

References for preparation

Unfortunately, no single book appears to cover all the knowledge and skills that are required for this paper. You need to be familiar with the basics of statistics and also understand the principles of critical appraisal and evidence-based medicine. The following list provides useful references for revision.

Useful texts for revision

- *Critical Reviews in Psychiatry*[4] (Papers and mock answers from the College).
- *How to Read a Paper*[5] (Critical appraisal methods).
- *How to Read a Paper*[6] (Series of articles).
- *How to Read a Paper*[7] (Internet versions of ref. 6).
- *Statistics with Confidence*[8] (A useful book for understanding confidence intervals).
- *A Practical Guide to Clinical Research in Psychiatry*[9] (A guide to research design for psychiatrists, with chapters on statistics).
- *Evidence Based Medicine*[10] (Critical appraisal methods).
- *Evidence-based Medicine*[11] (Detailed worked examples).
- *The Pocket Guide to Critical Appraisal*[12] (Excellent description of critical appraisal).
- *Evidence-based Mental Health.* BMJ Publishing Group, London (Short format papers with critical appraisal commentaries. See BMJ website (www.bmj.com) for internet version).
- Larger psychiatry textbooks also examine critical appraisal.

These will help you become familiar with the language of research and critical appraisal and should provide most of the answers to CRP questions.

The books in references 8–12 will enable you to answer most questions; however no single book summarises all the terms and definitions required. Because of this, Chapter 5 has been written to summarise key elements that are important for the exam. Particular attention is given to the need to understand specific scientific concepts with a numerical value, and how to calculate them. These concepts have precise definitions and it will be helpful during your revision to build up a list of these definitions.

Why has the College introduced this paper?

The College wants psychiatrists to learn critical appraisal skills. These skills underpin the growing trend towards evidence-based practice and the principle of lifelong learning. If you can read a paper and see its value, i.e. identify its good points and shortcomings, then you can assess that paper's relevance to your practice of psychiatry. You should make sure that your journal clubs become the main forum where you can practise critical appraisal skills with colleagues.

Knowledge and skills for the CRP

The syllabus and skills required are published in detail by the College. You will need to know about standard research methods. It is important to learn the advantages and disadvantages of the common study types. You also need a working knowledge of statistics. You must have an understanding of what standard statistical analyses can do and when they can be applied. Once you have appraised the methods and examined the analysis of data in a paper you should be able to assess the authors' conclusions. You should give a balanced answer, indicating strengths and weaknesses. At this point you can judge the relevance of the authors' work to your own practice and suggest ways of improving the design of the study.

Techniques for the CRP

You should start revision early. Critical review is a new area for many candidates, with an unfamiliar language. Not only are there novel ideas to learn in depth, but there are new terms to learn off by heart and associated numerical skills to develop. You will be expected to do calculations in the exam and you are allowed to take a simple non-programmable calculator in with you (make sure your calculator does not make beeping noises). Key terms are summarised in Chapter 5. You could compound errors too if terms such as the *likelihood ratio of a positive result* are calculated from the formula:

$$\frac{\text{sensitivity}}{(1-\text{specificity})}$$

– and you have previously calculated one of these values incorrectly. Early revision will give you time to familiarise yourself with the language of critical appraisal and practise the techniques.

Ring up for the College's information pack, sample papers and exam guidelines. Get a book of sample papers and answers to practise with. After your first attempt at a mock paper, make an assessment of your current abilities in critical review and begin to define the gaps in your knowledge. You can learn techniques for calculations such as the 2×2 table for screening test results (see worked example) which minimises confusion. Practise interpreting data in terms of the analytical definitions and calculations, e.g. *'How good is this anxiety test at picking out true cases?'* is the same as asking *'What is this anxiety test's sensitivity?'*, which is, numerically:

$$\frac{\text{(test positive true cases)}}{\text{(true cases)}}$$

Research methods

Different questions require different research methods. You need to know which method is best suited to each question. If you want to make conclusions about causation in the case of long-term exposure to environmental agents, you will need a different method to that used in assessing the effectiveness of a sleeping tablet. A description of the main research methods and common errors that may occur in research methodology are provided in Chapter 5.

You should be able to answer the following questions about any paper:

- Is the question relevant?
- Is the sampling satisfactory?
- Is the method appropriate to answer the question?
- Is the analysis appropriate and accurate?

- Are the results valid and reproducible?
- Has the question been answered definitively?
- Were there funding or ethical conflicts?
- Can and should I apply the findings in practice? Are the results generalisable?

The sampling procedure (and in particular whether the sample obtained is representative of the target population) is a key question. This is described in detail in Chapter 5.

Important questions to consider in your appraisal:

- What about the setting? Researchers in tertiary referral centres are unlikely to see the same patients as someone working within an inner city psychiatric sector.
- What about the selection of patients? What about exclusions/inclusions? How representative are they of the target population?
- How would you improve on the design?
- Are other methods of analysis indicated? Was the correct analysis carried out?
- Are missing patients properly accounted for (see CONSORT guidelines in Chapter 5).
- How would you address the limitations of this study in future work?

Be prepared to extend your criticism into positive steps towards more accurate studies and more definitive results.

Clinical relevance and clinical importance

Just because something is statistically significant does not mean that it is clinically important. Here is a list of the type of questions you may be asked about the paper under scrutiny:

- How would you use the results?

- How would you explain them to your patient?
- Would you use this drug? Is it safe?
- Would this test be applicable in a different setting (community/clinic/hospital)?
- Would you withdraw this treatment?

You can only answer such questions in an evidence-based fashion after critically appraising the type of study, the methods, analyses and strength of conclusions.

A comment on statistical tests

You need to know about the different forms of data such as **categorical** or **nominal** classifications (e.g. male or female). **Ordinal** data can be ranked in order of size (i.e. ordered). A regular scale, such as centigrade uses **interval** data. **Ratio** data have both a regular scale and also a true zero point (e.g. height in centimetres or temperature in degrees Kelvin).

Descriptive statistics

These include measures of central tendency such as the **mean** (average), **median** (middle value) and **mode** (most common result). Measures of spread include the **variance** (the mean of the sum of the squares of the difference from the mean), the **standard deviation** (the square root of the variance) and the **range** (the difference between the top and the bottom values). Measures of spread may have complex looking formulae which serve to turn inconvenient negative values into positive ones (by squaring them) and then make up for that by 'square rooting' them again. Details can be found in any book on statistics, or in Curran and Williams.[9]

The type of data distribution in your target population (not your sample population) determines which statistical tests you should use. When your target population data are evenly spread around the mean and the mean, median and mode are equal, the distribution curve is bell-shaped, and the distribution is called **normal** or **Gaussian**. This distribution has specific *parameters* and the statistics used when analysing data with such a distribution are called

parametric. Examples of normal distributions are height and weight in the general population. Non-normal or skewed data have asymmetrical distribution curves with unequal mean, median and mode. The significance tests for these populations do not have normal parameters and are called **non-parametric** or distribution-free tests.

Analytic statistics

Parametric statistics for normal data come in various forms. The simplest is the *t*-test. This can be an unpaired test for unrelated samples or a paired test if the samples are closely linked in some way (e.g. before and after comparisons on the same subjects). The test can be one- or two-tailed depending on whether you are interested in results in one or two directions. If you are only looking at the improvement brought about by a drug a one-tailed test is used, but if you want to examine improvement and deterioration, a two-tailed test would be appropriate. The *t* values can be looked up in tables which give probabilities (*p*-values) based on the sample size minus 1 (n–1) or *degrees of freedom*.

Non-parametric statistics include the Chi-squared test, Mann-Whitney U test for ordinal data and Wilcoxon tests. These are used for non-normal data and small samples. They tend to give less significant results than parametric tests and are often based on ranking of ordered data. It is tempting to use parametric statistics in preference to non-parametric, but if sample sizes are small or unlikely to be from a normally-distributed target population, parametric analysis would be inappropriate. Some researchers will **transform** their skewed data with a mathematical function, such as logarithms, to get around this.

Confidence intervals

These indicate the precision of the statistic calculated. They give a range rather then a cut-off. Confidence intervals (CIs) are like goal posts. If the goalkeeper is the calculated statistic, then the narrower the goal posts (CIs), the more confident you can be about the goalkeeper's effectiveness (i.e. to represent the true population value). Confidence intervals can be calculated for most statistics and are commonly used with sample means. For example, if you were comparing the average values of depression scale results in two samples and you calculated that the 95% CI of the difference in sample means of 10 was 5–15, this means that:

- there is a 95% chance that 5–15 includes the target population difference of means; or in more practical terms:
- 95% of identical studies would have a difference of means in the range 5–15.

Small samples with more spread (bigger standard errors) have wider confidence intervals and therefore give less precise results.

Evidence-based practice

There is little evidence yet that evidence-based medicine is widespread. A survey of 24 general practitioners revealed that they did not share the basic assumptions of evidence-based medicine and did not practise evidence-based medicine because of patient factors (co-morbidity and non-compliance) and lack of time, resources and skills. Observation of hospital specialist practice was just as likely to bring about changes of practice.[13] It may be reassuring to know that medical colleagues find critical appraisal difficult, but it also suggests that we should be as up to date as possible since, as specialists, we will be influencing the practice of others.

Critical review paper: worked example

Critical review can seem quite daunting. The worked example is also demanding and so a light-hearted scenario has been created to finish off this chapter.

> **Question**
>
> The examinations department recognised towards the end of the twentieth century that its examination system was causing candidates so much anxiety that a less stressful alternative was needed. Feedback from trainees highlighted the problems, which included months spent in revision, sleepless

nights in the week before examinations and profound gastrointestinal upsets on examination days.

After much debate the examinations department piloted a controversial new assessment based on the work of Rorschach which was first published in 1921. During a period of intensive research into early versions of the new assessment, candidates were sent four Rorschach inkblots and asked to jot down their general impressions of the images and return these in pre-paid envelopes. This paper reports a comparison of the inkblot results with the traditional exam results.

The results are presented here in a 2×2 table with the inner cells labelled by letter and the outer (totals) cells by letter sums. These are used in the calculation of test characteristics below. [Data are unlikely to be presented quite so helpfully in the exam but these tables can be constructed from the raw data of any dichotomous test that is compared with a dichotomous gold standard.]

		Traditional (gold standard) exam result		
		Pass	Fail	Totals
Results of inkblot test	Pass	a 82	b 93	$a+b = 175$
	Fail	c 7	d 18	$c+d = 25$
	Totals	$a+c = 89$	$b+d = 111$	$a+b+c+d = 200$

1. Comment on the rationale and methodology for this research.
2. (a) How good is the new assessment at identifying candidates who have passed the traditional exam? What is this aspect of a test called? Give its value.
   (b) How well does the new assessment identify candidates who have failed the traditional exam? What is this feature of a test called? Give its value.

3. Calculate the positive and negative predictive values and comment on the results.
4. What is the likelihood ratio for a positive result (i.e. a pass)?
5. Compare pre-test odds with post-test odds. (Alternatively compare pre- and post-test probabilities.)
6. Should the new test be introduced?

Answers

1. The research aims to find a satisfactory and less stressful alternative to the traditional examination. The new assessment is compared with the gold standard of the existing examination. The inkblot test is an observer-rated projective personality test. It is unlikely to measure the same things as the traditional exam. The test is subject to age, gender and cultural bias. No details of the method of interpretation are given. It is likely that the interpretation is qualitative rather than quantitative and inter-rater reliability between interpretations will be low. The omission of the methodology is a grave shortcoming in this research which means all the results are questionable. A 100% return rate is an excellent response rate and may be too good to be true.

2. The 2×2 table can be re-worked as:

		Traditional (gold standard) exam result			
		Pass	Fail	Totals	
Results of inkblot test	Pass	*a* 82	*b* 93	*a+b* = 175	**Positive predictive value = *a/(a+b)***
	Fail	*c* 7	*d* 18	*c+d* = 25	**Negative predictive value = *d/(c+d)***
	Totals	*a+c* = 89	*b +d* = 111	*a+b+c+d* = 200	
		Sensitivity = *a/(a+c)*	**Specificity = *d/(b+d)***		**Prevalence =*(a+c)/(a+b+c+d)***

(a) The test is good at identifying traditional exam passes. This aspect of a test is called the sensitivity. The proportion of traditional exam passes (gold standard) which are also new assessment passes is 92% ($a/(a+c)$ = 82/89).

(b) The test is poor at identifying candidates who failed the traditional exam. This feature of a test is called the specificity. The proportion of traditional exam failures which are also new assessment failures is 16% ($d/(b+d)$ = 18/111).

3. The positive predictive value is 47% ($a/(a+b)$ = 82/175). This is the proportion of new assessment passes which are also traditional exam passes. The negative predictive value is 72% ($d/(c+d)$ = 18/25). The new assessment is not a good indicator of the gold standard pass rate but is better at indicating a gold standard failure. (It is worth remembering that the positive predictive value is the same as the post-test probability of a pass).

4. The likelihood ratio for a pass is 1.1 (sensitivity/(1–specificity) = 0.92/(1–0.16)). The more extreme the likelihood ratio, the more useful the test. The least helpful tests have likelihood ratios of 1.

5. Pre-test odds = prevalence/(1–prevalence). The prevalence of gold standard passes is 45% (($a+c)/(a+b+c+d$) = 89/200). The pre-test odds are therefore 0.82 (0.45/0.55). Post-test odds = pre-test odds × likelihood ratio, which is 0.9 (0.82 ×1.1). The odds can be converted to probabilities with the formula: odds/(1+odds). So pre-test probability is 45% (0.82/1.82) and post-test probability is 47% (0.9/1.9) (which is the same as positive predictive value, above). The test gives us no further information than the prevalence alone and is therefore unhelpful.

6. The methodology is unclear and likely to be subject to many forms of bias. The results of the analysis are

suspect. The neutral likelihood ratio suggests the test would be unhelpful. The traditional exam has considerable face validity in that it examines candidates in the clinical process of history taking, mental state examination, and clinical decision making as well as theoretical background. The new assessment has no face validity and no theoretical rationale is given for the choice of the inkblot method. The new assessment should not be introduced and the traditional system with all its attendant stresses for candidates should be retained.

Key points

- Many aspects of the CRP are unfamiliar for many candidates.
- Start revision and mock papers early on in Part II preparation.
- Use journal clubs to practise critical appraisal.
- Collect together books and other resources to help you learn and revise.
- Create your own list of definitions and calculation formulae. **Use Chapter 5 to help you with this**.
- Learn about research methods, analyses and statistics.
- Get used to applying research to clinical practice.

REFERENCES

1. *MRCPsych Part II Guidance Notes*. Royal College of Psychiatrists, 17 Belgrave Square, London SW1X 8PG, UK. Tel: (020) 7235 2351.

2. *The Critical Review Paper Information Pack*. Royal College of Psychiatrists, 17 Belgrave Square, London SW1X 8PG, UK. Tel: (020) 7235 2351.

3. *The Basic Sciences and Clinical Curricula for the MRCPsych Examinations*. Royal College of Psychiatrists, 17 Belgrave Square, London SW1X 8PG, UK. Tel: (020) 7235 2351.

4. Brown T, Wilkinson G (1998) *Critical Reviews in Psychiatry*. Gaskell: London.

5. Greenhalgh T (1997) *How to Read a Paper.* BMJ Publishing Group: London.

6. Greenhalgh T (1997) How to read a paper. *British Medical Journal* 315: 243.

7. Greenhalgh T (1997) How to read a paper. Electronic *British Medical Journal* (www.bmj.com) 315: 243.

8. Gardner M, Altman D (1989) *Statistics with Confidence.* BMJ Books: London.

9. Curran S, Williams CJ (1999) *A Practical Guide to Clinical Research in Psychiatry.* Butterworth Heinemann: Oxford.

10. Sackett DL, Scott W, Richardson MD, Rosenberg W, Haynes RB (1996) *Evidence Based Medicine.* Churchill Livingstone: London.

11. Friedland DJ et al (1998) *Evidence-based Medicine.* Appleton & Lange: Stamford.

12. Crombie IK (1996) *The Pocket Guide to Critical Appraisal.* BMJ Books: London.

13. Tomlin Z, Humphrey C, Rogers S (1999) General practitioners' perceptions of effective health care. *British Medical Journal* 318: 1532–1535.

The critical review paper – key topics for revision

Catherine Brown

Introduction

Chapter outline

This chapter will summarise:

- Types of data
- Common statistical tests
- Definitions of some important statistical terms
- Screening and diagnosis
- Randomised controlled trials (RCTs)
- Case control/cohort studies
- Systematic reviews and meta-analysis.

Candidates approaching the critical review paper need to know and understand the key concepts of how to carry out effective critical appraisal. The concepts of critical appraisal are summarised in a number of good books (e.g. Crombie[1]). However, many of the key statistical concepts required are not covered well from any one source and are therefore particularly difficult to learn for the purpose of the exam. This chapter is not meant to be a comprehensive account of all that is required for the critical review paper; however, it does aim to provide explanations and definitions for some of the terms and phrases that candidates often have difficulty with. Basic statistics (e.g. calculating the mean, median and mode) have not been included. A clear description of these and more advanced tests can be found within Curran and Williams.[2] It is important to realise that learning these definitions by rote is not enough. You must attempt to **understand** these concepts which are drawn from the fields of research design and methodology, statistics and critical appraisal. Read about the different definitions and terms using different sources and practise applying them to the papers that you read in order to reinforce your learning.

Types of data

Type of data	Nominal	Ordinal	Interval	Ratio
Categories mutually exclusive	×	×	×	×
Categories logically ordered		×	×	×
Equal distance between adjacent categories			×	×
True zero point				×

Common statistical tests

Descriptive statistics

Mean, standard deviation. Median, mode, range.

Analytical statistics

	Parametric	Non-parametric
Comparison of two groups	Students *t*-test (paired or independent/unpaired)	a) 2 independent groups: Mann-Whitney U Test b) Paired data: Wilcoxon rank sum test
Compare a large number of groups	ANOVA	Kruskal-Wallis ANOVA
Correlation coefficients (looking for an association between two variables)	Pearson correlation coefficient	Spearman rank correlation coefficient
Multivariate analysis	MANOVA Multiple regression Logistic regression	

Standard deviation

- The spread of all the observations around the mean.
- Calculated as *square root of the variance.*
- Have the same units as the original observations.

$$sd = \sqrt{\Sigma \frac{(x - \bar{x})^2}{n - 1}}$$

sd = the square root of the variance, hence the variance = sd^2.

- In a normal (Gaussian) distribution:

  67% of the values lie between +/– 1 sd
  95% of the values lie between +/– 2 sd
  99% of the values lie between +/– 3 sd.

Standard error

The standard error = standard deviation/$\sqrt{n}$ and hence includes a measure of sample size.

- It reflects the variability of the mean of the sample as an estimate of the true mean of the general population from which the sample was taken.

ANOVA (analysis of variance)

- Compares the variability of observations around the mean within a group to the variability between group means.
- Can identify big differences but not where they lie.
- Needs further post-hoc tests to identify where these differences lie (e.g. *t*-tests; Scheffe test to examine the possible combinations of group means).

Correlation coefficients

- Degree of annotation/association between observations. Rated 0 = no association, to 1 (or –1), directly (or inversely) associated.
- Describe average relationships.
- Cannot discuss cause and effect (e.g. smoking and lung cancer).
- Prone to confounding – other factors may have led to the finding.

Multiple regression

- A measure of association is calculated taking a number of confounders (e.g. age, sex) into account simultaneously.
- A form of multivariate analysis.
- Applies when the dependent variable is continuous.

Logistic regression

- Used when the dependent variable is binary/dichotomous.
- The risk of developing an outcome is expressed as a function of independent predictor variables.
- The dependent variable is defined as **the natural log of the odds of the disease**.
- Can be converted to an odds ratio (see later) that is adjusted for confounding and/or into '**product terms**' to assess interactions.

Cox-proportional hazards/regression

- A method for modelling time-to-event data. The Cox regression allows you to include predictor variables (covariates) in your models (e.g. '*Do men and women have different risks of developing lung cancer based on cigarette smoking?*'). By constructing a Cox regression model with cigarette usage (cigarettes smoked per day) and gender entered as covariates, you can test hypotheses regarding the effects of gender and cigarette usage on time-to-onset for lung cancer'. (Definition and example taken from SPSS for Windows, version 8.)
- Includes a time factor – appropriate if subjects have not been followed up for an equal length of time.
- Another statistical approach used within survival analysis is the **Kaplan Meier survival analysis**.

Definitions of some important statistical terms

Target population

- The target population makes up a large pool of information from which we draw a proportion for study (sample population, see below). It will contain every eligible person or item having the characteristics of interest.

Sample population

- The sample population is a collection of individuals or items taken from a target population. The aim is for the sample population to be **representative** of the target population so that any conclusions drawn from the sample population can have **validity** and **generalisability**. Methods of sampling include random sampling, stratified random sampling, multi-stage random sampling and cluster sampling. Badly chosen samples can result in **selection bias**.

Null hypothesis

- The null hypothesis (sometimes called H_0) assumes that there is no effect (no difference) between the experimental and control groups, i.e. the data have come from a chance-based distribution.
- This contrasts with the experimental hypothesis (H_1) that assumes there is a true difference between the groups that has **not** arisen by chance.

Statistical significance

- Conventionally used to indicate the likelihood of a result as, or more, extreme than what is found, had it been drawn from a chance-based distribution (i.e. the probability of it occurring by **chance**).

p value

- If the null hypothesis were true, *p* is the probability of getting your result or a more extreme value by chance.
- If *p* is very small (conventionally taken as $p \leq 0.05$ or smaller), any difference observed is judged to have been unlikely to have occurred by chance. Thus the null hypothesis can be rejected – there **is** a difference between groups.

Clinical significance

Just because a result is statistically significant does not mean that the difference observed is of sufficient magnitude to be apparent and important in a **clinical** setting, i.e. is it of **clinical significance** rather than merely statistical significance?

Confidence intervals (CIs)

- The range of values within which we can be 95% sure (or whatever CI level is chosen) that the true value lies for the target population from whom the study patients were selected.
- If a series of identical studies were carried out repeatedly on different samples from the same population, then 95% results would lie between these values.
- Tells us about the strength of the evidence rather than if there is just a difference.
- It provides all the information of the *p* value **plus** it also takes into account sample size.
- Expressed in units of whatever the confidence interval applies to.

Bias

Bias is 'any process at any stage of inference which tends to produce results or conclusions that differ from the truth' (Sackett[3]).

Sources of bias in primary studies

- **Selection bias** – the subjects selected to be in the study (i.e. the sample population) may be different in some way from the population you aim to investigate.
- **Subject bias** – if the subject knows they are being observed or tested in some way they may behave differently to how they would normally.
- **Observer bias** – if the observer is aware of the aim of the study, the hypothesis being tested or whether the subject is in a treatment or control group, their assessment of the characteristics of interest may be biased. Sometimes this can be overcome by making sure the assessor is blind to allocation but this is not always possible.
- **Recall bias** – this may occur in retrospective studies, e.g. case-control studies when there is a difference in knowledge between subjects in the case and control groups leading to a biased recall. For example 'cases' may more readily recall exposure to a particular agent which may be associated with a disease than the 'controls'.

> - **Information bias** – includes observer and recall bias.
> - **Confounding bias** – occurs when a confounding factor is associated with both the suspected risk factor and the disorder.

Confounding variables/factors

- Should always be considered in interpreting results, especially non-randomised or observational studies.

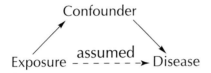

- These are associated with both the outcome of a study and the independent variables of interest (the exposure).
- Confounders have more influence upon outcome than the independent variables.

Type I error

- Occurs when the null hypothesis is rejected even though it is true.
- A statistical difference is found between two groups even though no true difference exists.
- Also called a **false positive** result.
- The probability of making a Type I error is equal to the *p* value and expressed as alpha (α – typically set at 0.05).
- Reasons for Type I errors are bias and confounding.

Type II error

- Occurs when the null hypothesis is accepted whereas the null hypothesis is in fact false.
- The study failed to detect a true difference between groups.
- A **false negative** result.
- Represented by beta (β – typically set at 0.2).
- Related to the **power** of the study.

Power

- Probability of rejecting the null hypothesis when a true difference exists.

- Represented by $(1-\beta) = 0.8$ or 80% power – the level normally seen as acceptable.
- Complex relationship dependent upon:
  - sample size
  - size of effect
  - reliability of measures
  - adopted significance level.
- Therefore adequate power is achieved by:
  - large sample size
  - large effect sizes
  - high reliability
  - 0.05 significance level.

Screening and diagnosis

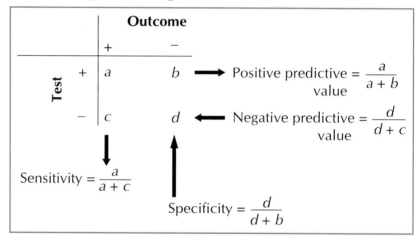

Sensitivity

- Ability to diagnose disease when present.
- **Probability of diagnosing disease when present**.
- Those who have the outcome/disease that are correctly identified as positive by the test.

Specificity

- Ability to identify absence of disease when disease is not present.
- **Probability of not diagnosing the disease when absent**.

- Those who do not have outcome/disease that are correctly identified as negative by the test.

Positive predictive value (PPV)
- The proportion of individuals who are identified as positive on the test **who are in fact** positive (have the disease/outcome).

Negative predictive value (NPV)
- The proportion of individuals identified as negative by the test **who are in fact** negative (do not have the disease/outcome).

Likelihood ratio for a positive result
- $\dfrac{\text{sensitivity}}{(1 - \text{specificity})}$ $\quad$ (true positives) / (false positives)

- The likelihood that a positive test result will be observed in a patient as opposed to one without the disorder.
- Many reports of diagnostic tests provide multilevel likelihood ratios as measures of their accuracy.

Likelihood ratio for a negative result
- $\dfrac{(1 - \text{sensitivity})}{\text{specificity}}$ $\quad$ (false negatives) / (true negatives)

Pre-test odds
- $\dfrac{\text{prevalence}}{(1 - \text{prevalence})} = \dfrac{\dfrac{(a + c)}{(a + b + c + d)}}{1 - \dfrac{(a + c)}{(a + b + c + d)}}$

Post-test odds
- Pre-test odds × likelihood ratio.

Post-test probability
- $\dfrac{\text{post-test odds}}{(\text{post-test odds} + 1)}$ $\quad$ (converts odds to risk)

Pre-test probability

- Same as prevalence = $\dfrac{(a + c)}{(a + b + c + d)}$

Key points

- Remember risk (probability) $= \dfrac{\text{odds}}{(1 + \text{odds})}$ and odds $= \dfrac{\text{risk}}{(1 - \text{risk})}$

Nomogram

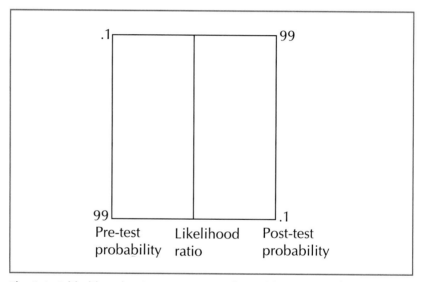

Fig. 5.1 A likelihood ratio nomogram. Adapted from Fagan, [4] as used in Sackett et al.[5]

A nomogram can be used to interpret diagnostic test results, to help you decide whether a diagnostic test produces important changes from pre-test to post-test probabilities.

Reliability

- Relates to the level of agreement between repeated measurements.
- Implies diagnostic consistency.

Measures of reliability

- **Inter-rater** – the level of agreement between assessments of the same material made by two or more assessors at roughly the same time.
- **Intra-rater** – the level of agreement between assessments of the same material made by the same assessor at two or more different times (with videoed or tape recorded material).
- **Test–re-test** – the level of agreement or correlation between repeat administration of the test under similar circumstances.
- **Alternative forms** – two forms of the same test are created and administered at the same time or consecutively.
- **Split half** – the test or measurement is administered, split in half then the scores on one half are correlated with the other half.
- Statistical tests of reliability:
  - percentage agreement
  - product moment correlation coefficient
  - kappa statistic
  - intra-class correlation coefficient.

Validity

- Term used to determine whether a particular test measures what it aims to measure. The extent to which it corresponds to a 'gold standard' or how well diagnoses compare to external validators (e.g. concurrent symptoms, cause of illness, diagnostic stability, biological markers, familial pattern, response to treatment).
- Validity is dependent on reliability.

Types of validity

- **Face validity** – on the surface does the test appear to be measuring what you are trying to measure? Not strictly a true type of validity.
- **Content validity** – similar concept but less superficial. Do the specific measurements aimed for by the

---

instrument assess the content of the measurement in question?

- **Predictive (prognostic) validity** – the extent of agreement between the test and a test in the future or predicted outcome.
- **Concurrent validity** – how does the test compare to already existing established tests or some sort of external validator?
- **Criterion validity** – predictive and concurrent validity are sometimes referred to together as criterion validity.
- **Incremental validity** – is the test/measure superior to other measures in approaching true validity?
- **Cross validity** – after a test has been criterion validated on one sample does it maintain criterion validity when applied to another sample?
- **Convergent validity** – do different measures of the same construct produce the same outcome and are they correlated?
- **Divergent validity** – does the test discriminate between other measures of unrelated constructs?
- **Construct validity** – constructs are abstract concepts and difficult to measure directly. Construct validity includes convergent and divergent validity and is connected with the underlying theory which is the basis of the test/instrument.

Randomised controlled trials (RCTs)

What is a randomised control trial?

- A trial in which subjects are randomly assigned to two or more groups (i.e. have an equal chance of being allocated to any group).
- The experimental group receives the intervention that is being tested.
- The comparison or control groups receive alternative treatments.
- The groups are followed up to see if any differences are evident, which can then be attributed to the new intervention.

CONSORT guidelines (Altman[6])

- All patients assessed for the trial should be accounted for plus the report should be accompanied by a guideline that explains what happened to all the patients involved in the trial.
- The randomisation procedure should be clearly specified.
- Inclusion plus exclusion criteria should be clearly stated.
- The method of blinding should be specified.
- There should be an **intention to treat** analysis.

Randomisation

- A procedure that ensures all subjects recruited to a trial have an equal chance of being allocated to the treatment or control groups.
- The purpose is to eliminate the **bias** which occurs when experimenters are allowed to influence subject allocation.
- The aim is to provide two or more identical groups of patients so that any differences observed can be attributed to the different treatments.
- Potentially **confounding** variables should be evenly distributed throughout the randomised groups.
- If there are known confounders (e.g. age), sometimes stratification is used.
- The gold standard method of randomisation is the production of a **computer generated random number** at a **site distant from study** done by an **independent person** with good **concealment**.

Power calculation

- This is used to determine how many subjects are required for a clinical trial to have a good chance of detecting a clinically significant difference on a particular outcome variable – **if there is a difference**.

- $$\dfrac{\text{Clinically significant difference}}{\text{sd}} \longrightarrow \text{table of power for given number of subjects}$$

80% power is the generally accepted cut-off $(1-\beta)$ (β = Type II error).

Intention to treat analysis

- Data on all randomised subjects are analysed within the groups to which they were assigned.
- Any other policy towards dropouts will involve subjective decisions, plus will create an opportunity for bias.

- Drop outs are an important group and therefore must be included. This group is relevant to clinical practice ('real life').

Informed consent

- The patient should understand the nature and purpose of the study and any risks and benefits of the intervention/treatment.
- The patient should understand that if they refuse to participate, normal treatment will not be affected.
- They should know that they can withdraw at any time without giving a reason and without affecting their treatment.
- They should know they have an equal chance of being allocated to control and treatment groups.
- The explanation should be given orally and in writing. They should have time to consider before deciding.
- A detailed discussion of research ethics and design is provided in Prothero.[7]

Blinding

May mean:

- The patient is unaware whether they are in the treatment or control group
- The therapist/investigator is unaware of group allocation
- Both (**double blind**) – the strongest research design.

Common problems in RCTs

If you know a list of problems in all RCTs you can apply these to a specific paper in the exam:

- Failures of true randomisation
- Inadequate concealment
- Lack of blind treatment or outcome assessment
- Ignoring missing data
- Inappropriate and/or too many outcome measures
- Patients likely to give informed consent and participate in the trial are often different from the 'average' patient. For example, in psychiatry, patients with more than one diagnosis or concurrent substance abuse are often excluded from RCTs).
- The development of **pragmatic trials** aims to overcome some of these criticisms.

Experimental event rate (EER)

- The rate of a dichotomous outcome in the group receiving the new intervention.
- Event may be positive (e.g. recovery) or negative (e.g. drop outs/side effects, etc.).
- Can be expressed as % or fraction.

Control event rate (CER)

- The rate of dichotomous outcome in the group receiving control or standard intervention.

Relative risk reduction (RRR)

- The proportional reduction in event rates between the treatment groups:

$$\frac{CER - EER}{EER}$$

Absolute risk reduction (ARR)

- Absolute difference in event rates in exceptional and control groups.

$$EER - CER = ARR \text{ (expressed as \% or fraction)}.$$

Number needed to treat (NNT)

- Clinically useful measure of a treatment's value.
- The number of people one needs to treat with a specific intervention to achieve one **additional** favourable outcome.
- Calculated by: $\dfrac{1}{ARR}$

Effect size

- Often reported in terms of sd units or odds ratio.
- $\dfrac{\text{Difference between two means}}{\text{Standard deviation}}$ (Cohen's *d*) (standardised difference)
- Numerically equivalent to *z* scores.

Case control and cohort studies

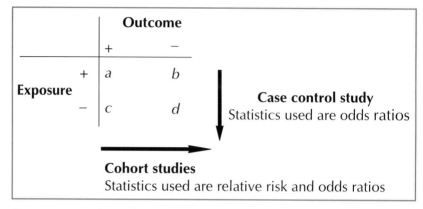

Case control study

- Usually retrospective but can also be prospective, cross-sectional and longitudinal.
- May be only way to investigate a **rare** disease/outcome.
- Controls should come from the same population as the cases but not have the disease.
- Can only demonstrate **association**, not causation.

Example:

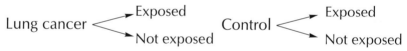

Cohort study

- Prospective.
- (Ideally) an **inception cohort** is followed up over time and outcome assessed.
- Can take years (e.g. decades).

Example:

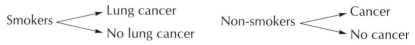

Probability

- The likelihood of any event occurring relative to (as a proportion of) the total number of possibilities. For example, in a drawer of red and green socks only, the probability of picking a green sock will be:

$$\frac{\text{no. of green socks}}{(\text{no. of green socks + no. of red socks})}$$

- Probability = risk.

Odds

- The odds of picking a green sock would be:

$$\frac{\text{no. of green socks}}{\text{no. of red socks}}$$

Converting risk to odds:

$$\text{Risk} = \frac{\text{odds}}{(1 + \text{odds})} \qquad \text{odds} = \frac{\text{risk}}{(1 - \text{risk})}$$

Odds ratio

- A measure of the strength of a treatment effect or an aetiological association, calculated by comparing outcome rates in exposed and non-exposed patients.
- The ratio of odds of an outcome in the experimental group, divided by the odds of an outcome in the other group.

$$\bullet \quad \frac{\text{Odds of exposure if have the disease/outcome}}{\text{Odds of exposure if don't have the disease/outcome}} = \frac{a/c}{b/d} = \frac{ad}{bc}$$

$$\bullet \quad \frac{\text{Odds of disease/outcome if exposed}}{\text{Odds of disease/outcome if not exposed}} = \frac{a/b}{c/d} = \frac{ad}{bc}$$

Relative risk

- The ratio of risk of outcome in one experimental group divided by risk of outcome in the other group.

$$\bullet \quad \frac{\text{Incidence in those exposed}}{\text{Incidence in those not exposed}} = \frac{a/a + b}{c/c + d} = \frac{a\,(c + d)}{c\,(a + b)}$$

Why calculate the odds ratio?

- You cannot calculate relative risk in case-control studies because you have no information about incidence.
- But if the disease is rare and the incidence is small, the odds ratio approximates to relative risk. Therefore in these cases it is useful to calculate the odds ratio.
- Statistically this is because:

$$ RR = \frac{a\,(c + d)}{c\,(a + b)} \longrightarrow \approx \frac{ad}{bc} $$

If disease is rare a and c are relatively small numbers.

Systematic reviews and meta-analysis

Systematic reviews

- Pre-specify types of article to be included and excluded.
- Use specific search strategies to identify relevant articles.
- Cite all identified articles.
- Have some system for measuring quality of different studies.
- A detailed description of the process of carrying out a systematic review is given in Glanville.[8]

Meta-analysis

- Individual trials often have different or conflicting results.
- 'Rate counting' techniques do not assess quality and have lower power.
- Meta-analyses derive a quantitative summary of effect size by statistically combining effect sizes weighted by study size/quality.
- They can be non-systematic.
- They cannot combine non-randomised trials with RCTs.
- They are sensitive to:
    - **publication** bias
    - **location** bias
    - **inclusion** bias.[9]

- They are influenced by the quality of the original trials.
- They are unreliable if event rates are low and number of studies small.
- They may give unreliable precision in observation studies.
- They may disagree with results from the largest RCT.

Publication bias

- The tendency for researchers to only write up and submit research with a positive result.
- Tendency for journals to accept and publish articles with a positive result.
- More evident in observational and intervention studies.
- Often associated with other types of bias; it is important to evaluate and control for this bias.

Location bias

- Language (e.g. omit foreign language journals in a systematic review).
- Database (only examine certain abstracting databases such as Medline and omit a significant part of the relevant literature as a result).
- Citation (mention only studies identified by others).
- Multiple publication (the same data presented as if it represents more than one study).

Inclusion bias

- Bias may arise in establishing the inclusion criteria for a meta-analysis.
- If the inclusion criteria are developed by an investigator familiar with the field of study the criteria may be influenced by the knowledge of the results of the potential studies.[9]

Heterogeneity

- Heterogeneity is a systematic difference in the effects in different studies beyond that expected by chance.
- Substantial heterogeneity between studies can bias the summary effect and may reflect important methodological differences and/or mean there are different sub-groups of patients, therefore it is important to identify this bias.

- Methods of testing heterogeneity:
  - 'eyeball' **funnel plot**
  - calculate **Q statistic**
  - **Galbraith plot** (identifies which studies contribute most to heterogeneity).

Summary estimates and calculation

- Meta-analysis calculates **summary effect size** (odds ratio) by taking the mean of all the individual study effect sizes 'weighted' by the individual study size.
- Weighting is done according to standard error either by:
  - **fixed effects modelling**: assumes each study is an estimate of a single underlying effect (i.e. favours large studies)
  - **random effects modelling**: assumes all studies included are a true random sample of all studies.

Other types of studies to know about

- Surveys.
- Single case studies.
- Qualitative studies.
- Economic analysis.

> **Key points**
> - Read certain key texts concerning critical appraisal and research methodology (e.g. Crombie,[1] Sackett et al,[5] Curran and Williams.[2]
> - Statistical and research definitions are often defined in a number of books. Use the current chapter to help identify areas that you should both understand and be able to define.
> - Learning the definitions by rote is not enough. You must attempt to **understand the concepts** involved.
> - Read about the different definitions and terms using different sources and practise applying them to the papers that you read in order to reinforce your learning.

Acknowledgements
We wish to thank Helen Prince for her helpful comments on this chapter.

REFERENCES

1. Crombie IK (1996) *The Pocket Guide to Critical Appraisal.* BMJ Books: London.

2. Curran S, Williams CJ (1999) *A Practical Guide to Clinical Research in Psychiatry.* Butterworth Heinemann: Oxford.

3. Sackett DL (1979) Bias in analytic research. *Journal of Chronic Disease* 32: 51–63. Taken from: Johnstone EC, Freeman CPL, Zealley AK (1990) *Companion to Psychiatric Studies,* Sixth Edition. Churchill Livingstone: London.

4. Fagan TJ (1975) Nomogram from Bayes's theorem (c). *New England Journal of Medicine* 293: 257.

5. Sackett DL, Scott W, Richardson MD, Rosenberg W, Haynes RB (1996) *Evidence Based Medicine.* Churchill Livingstone: London.

6. Altman AG (1996) Better reporting of randomised controlled trials: the CONSORT statement. *British Medical Journal* 313: 570–571.

7. Prothero A (1999) Ethical issues in research. In: Curran S, Williams CJ (1999) *A Practical Guide to Clinical Research in Psychiatry.* Butterworth Heinemann: Oxford.

8. Glanville J (1999) Carrying out the literature search. In: Curran S, Williams CJ (1999) *A Practical Guide to Clinical Research in Psychiatry.* Butterworth Heinemann: Oxford.

9. Egger M, Davey Smith G (1990) Meta-analysis bias in location and selection of studies. *British Medical Journal* 316: 61–66.

OTHER USEFUL REFERENCES

• Bowers D (1996) *Statistics from Scratch. An Introduction for Health Care Professionals.* Wiley & Sons: Chichester.

• Puri BK, Tyrer PJ (1998) *Sciences Basic to Psychiatry.* Churchill Livingstone: Edinburgh.

• Hall AD, Puri BK (1997) *Revision Notes in Psychiatry.* Arnold: London.

Essay technique

David Yeomans

The Part II exam includes an essay paper which lasts 90 minutes. Candidates are required to answer one from two questions on 'General Psychiatry' and one from two on 'Psychiatric Specialties'.

Possible essay topics

General psychiatry questions may cover a surprising range of topics:

- Clinical
- Epidemiology
- Diagnostic systems
- Need for psychiatric services/ setting up services
- Rehabilitation
- Transcultural psychiatry
- Hospital liaison
- Neuropsychiatry
- HIV
- Medicine relevant to psychiatry
- Research.

Psychiatric specialties questions may include:
- Child and adolescent
- Forensic
- Mental handicap
- Psychiatry of old age
- Psychotherapy.

63

Preparation

When you draw up your revision timetable be sure to set aside regular time to practise essays. Writing is physically tiring and is a skill that you may not have practised for several years. By the end of your revision you should have written 10–20 essay plans and at least two full length pieces.

Reading is your major source of factual information. You cannot read everything, so be selective:

- Review articles in major journals (e.g. *British Journal of Psychiatry*) and review journals (e.g. *Current Opinion*) are useful. Read the exam syllabus in the *Inceptors Handbook* (from Royal College of Psychiatrists) to see which areas you need to know and which you don't. Send off for past papers and obtain the most recent exam papers from colleagues who have recently taken the exam
- Work out what major topics you wish to cover. Many candidates find it useful to produce a collection of 'essay plans'. If you prepare 15–20 topics, some of them may be included in the actual exam.

Essay spotting

There are several assumptions underlying the technique of essay spotting:

- Certain topics are important and these tend to be repeated
- If such a topic has not come up recently then the chances of it appearing as a question in the next exam may be increased
- Currently topical issues may be set on the essay paper (e.g. nation-wide changes in service provision, Mental Health Act, prominent review articles). Look at the editorials and reviews that have appeared in the last 12 months of the *Psychiatric Bulletin* and the *British Journal of Psychiatry.*

The choice of essays on the paper is very limited (currently one from two on each section of the essay paper). As a result, some candidates may immediately discount the possibility of being able to answer **any** of the questions at all. If you concentrate on using effective essay technique during your preparation and on the day of the exam, however, you will be able to make a good attempt at writing the two essays required. On first seeing the paper, do not automatically discount **any** of the questions. **Stop and think** how you might answer each question before making your choice.

The techniques outlined in this chapter can put you at an advantage over other candidates who will not have practised these techniques, let alone written an essay for many years.

Structuring an essay

What is an essay? It is a long written piece held together by a **structure** and contains **arguments** supported by **information**. A common structure for an essay is an **introduction**, then the **arguments**, followed by your **conclusion**. This basic structure may need to be modified depending on how the essay question is asked. A very open question such as 'Describe the uses of medical audit' requires you to define the structure yourself. A question such as 'Discuss the effects of antidepressants on the course and outcome of anxiety disorders' is more clearly defined, but you must still impose some structure on your answer. This can be done using the techniques described below.

- Spend a few minutes before you start writing to prepare an **essay plan**. Write out your essay structure at the beginning of the essay and label it as the essay outline. You can then refer back to it as you write in order to maintain the structure and keep track of the remaining time. Cross out those areas you have covered so that you can see how the essay is progressing. Take time to review the content intermittently in case any fresh ideas come to mind.
- Six useful questions are: **Who? What? Why? Where? When? How?** When tackling the essay, ask yourself these questions to help produce a critical discussion.

Think about what terms the question uses. **What** is medical audit? **Who** is interested in audit? **Why** should doctors get involved? **How** is anxiety defined? **How many** different antidepressants are there? **What** is outcome? **How** is it measured?

- **Helicoptering**. A helicopter can hover miles up in the sky to obtain a broad view of the situation. It can descend to various points in that landscape to see more details. You can do this in an essay by alternating between a general overview and more focused and detailed argument.

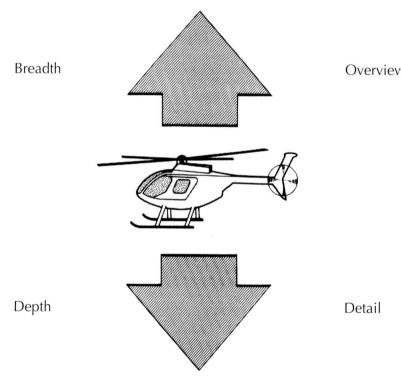

Fig 6.1 Helicoptering.

Expansion techniques

Before setting pen to paper expand the question to its limits by considering all the subject areas you can include. Helpful sub-headings to expand the scope of your thinking (and hence your essay) include:

- Biological, psychological and social aspects
- Acute, intermediate and long term
- Male and female differences
- Age differences
- Cultural differences
- Approaching the question from the point of view of different sub-specialties (such as child psychiatry, psychiatry of the elderly, liaison psychiatry, etc.)
- 'Non medical' factors such as the impact on carers, media influences, politics, and finance
- Past, present and future implications.

Worked example 1

Candidates on the Leeds MRCPsych Part II Examination Techniques course were asked to use the above techniques to create essay plans. Although no one felt prepared for the task, one group produced the following essay structure within 10 minutes.

Question

Discuss medical classification and how it has been applied in psychiatry.

Answer

INTRODUCTION: Why is classification necessary?
- Communication
- Universal use
- Predict prognosis
- It aids research so that different researchers can study similar patients
- Implications for treatment

CLASSIFICATION METHODS
- Syndromal: grouping of symptoms and signs

- Aetiology: infective, trauma, genetic, etc.
- Course: acute, chronic or remitting
- Outcome
- Multi-axial definitions (or a combined biopsychosocial model)

APPLICATION OF CLASSIFICATION MODELS IN PSYCHIATRY

- The current systems: ICD, DSM
- Lack of success, lack of clear aetiologies and the limitations of syndromal classification
- Outcome predictions are actually quite poor
- Historical perspective: e.g. Kraepelin

CONCLUSIONS

- Slow but steady progress is being made
- More consensus than before
- Future hope to include more aetiological and pathological data with multi-axial descriptions taken into account

This essay structure demonstrates some of the techniques described above. First of all, you **must read the question in full**. A simple approach with an introduction, arguments, and conclusion is used. There is a clear structure. The candidates in this case defined **what** classification is and **why** it is used. They focused down from the two broad questions on classification and application and split each up into several headings. For some of the headings they focused down further to give detailed examples which illustrate the benefits and pitfalls of using diagnostic systems. They then 'helicoptered' up again to allow a wider discussion of the arguments. The essay structure is **critical** and asks **how successful** classification is in psychiatry. It looks to **what** the future may hold and expands the question a little beyond what was asked. Perhaps it could have included some consideration of cultural differences and similarities. You may already have different ideas of how you would answer this question. Why not try them out now?

Worked example 2

> ## Question
> *How can exploratory psychotherapy lead to a worsening of a patient's condition? What can be done to reduce this?*
>
> ## Answer
> ### INTRODUCTION
>
> Definitions:
> **(a)** **Exploratory psychotherapy:** dynamic psychotherapy; types/methods; individual/group/family; in children and adults
> **(b)** **Worsening:**
> > **(i)** In therapy: transference/counter-transference issues; risks of dependency
> > **(ii)** Out of therapy: acting out; also to consider problems in work or with their family
> > **(iii)** General: risks of parasuicide/self-harm; anxiety or depression
>
> ### ARGUMENTS
> These went on to discuss the above ideas, and particularly to discuss the 'worsening' in terms of overall outcome
>
> ### WHAT CAN BE DONE TO PREVENT WORSENING?
> - Patient selection including liaison with referrers
> - Training and supervision of psychotherapists
> - Conjoint work and treatment (e.g. additional medication from general practitioners)
> - The importance of clear communication and continuity of treatment
> - Monitor the mental state closely
> - Assess defence mechanisms for potential vulnerability to psychological treatment approaches
> - Pay attention to transference and counter-transference issues and difficulties

- Give adequate preparation for times of absence by the therapist
- Consider the frequency of sessions and the risks of dependency occurring

The candidates' reaction to this essay title was interesting. Initially they felt great pessimism when given this question to attempt. They said that they would never have chosen this topic in an exam, and believed that they would answer it very badly because they did not have any specialised expertise in this field. None expected to produce such an extensive outline until they applied the techniques taught above. They were surprised to find out exactly how much they really knew. Had this been the only question they could remotely hope to answer, this technique-based approach would have given them a much better chance of success.

The role of the examiner

The examiner has to mark multiple essays on the same question. Remember he or she may well be bored and would prefer to be doing something else. It is your task to present them with a clearly legible, well written, structured essay that stands out from all the others.

What to do

The instructions on the exam paper state:

> The answers should be written in *essay form*; in addition, tables and/or diagrams may be used wherever these add to the clarity of the candidate's account. The candidate is expected to communicate clearly, present arguments coherently, evaluate evidence and make balanced judgements. The answers should refer to the basic scientific, as well as clinical, aspects of each topic. Extra marks will be given for appropriate and critical reference to the literature and research findings. **Illegibility will be penalised**.

> Source: Royal College of Psychiatrists Examination Paper, 1999. Royal College of Psychiatrists, Belgrave Square, London.

Candidates who do not take these instructions seriously, particularly regarding legibility of handwriting, will have much greater difficulty in passing the exam.

Important guidelines

- Write legibly.
- Consider writing double-spaced. This makes your essay easier on the eye and simpler to mark.
- Break up the text with headings, lists, diagrams and tables where appropriate. (Take a look at your textbooks and see how they present information. Each chapter in the book is itself an essay.)
- Use colour (e.g. a red pen) to highlight important points or sub-headings using underlining.
- Provide references where possible (name and year if you can, if not, state what you can remember, e.g. 'A paper published in the British Journal of Psychiatry last month showed . . .').
- Write naturally, but consider the following. Short sentences add impact. Long sentences with no punctuation such as commas that go on for line after line and talk about different subjects without so much as a pause between them do tend to confuse and the examiner does not want to re-read the essay 10 times to work out what you are trying to say. See?
- Show the examiners that you can order information, and make the presentation and structure clear by the use of sub-headings.
- Bullet points can be very effective in lists.

What <u>not</u> to do

Don't make things up. Don't waffle about irrelevancies. Do not write about a totally different question just because you have prepared an essay plan about it. You will get no marks unless you answer the question that is asked. Remember this point when you have 'spotted' a question. You need to tailor the prepared answer to the question on the exam paper. Do not be unbalanced in your arguments. Remember that your essay reveals things about you. Examiners may be concerned if, for example, you appear to have no consideration for patients' well being. Finally, remember that an essay requires a reasonably lengthy piece of writing – one page is not enough!

What are your blindspots?

When you write a practice essay, ask someone to comment critically about it. You may be unaware of habitual spelling or grammatical errors. You may not notice a tendency to leave words unfinished (one of the authors has this proble). Let someone else discover your blindspots, but be critical of **their** criticism. In the end you have to rely on your own style.

Key points

- Read the questions carefully and answer the question you have been asked.
- Answers should be written in essay form. You should communicate clearly, present coherent arguments, evaluate evidence and produce balanced judgements.
- Structure your answer clearly. Illegibility will be penalised.
- Use helicoptering to produce a broad overview and then focus on specific areas.
- Use questions such as **Why? What? Where? When? How?** Take on different perspectives (child, adult, old age, etc.) to keep your answer broad.
- Use expansion techniques.
- Gain extra points by using reference to the literature.

Preparing for the long case

Christopher Williams

The long case clinical examination occurs in both the Part I and Part II exams. At present, to pass overall, you **must** be successful in the long case. How can you stand out as being someone who should pass? The general principles of doing well in the clinical exams are to organise your knowledge, making what you say:

- Clear
- Relevant
- Interesting.

Remember:

- Clear communicators consistently do well.
- You are presenting **yourself**, not merely the case.
- It is not a test of detailed academic knowledge; this is covered in the written papers.
- You are also being asked to demonstrate your skills as a clinician.

You need to demonstrate to the examiners that you are a safe, sensible and competent clinician who could be trusted to look after their patients.

Preparation

The good news is that you know in advance what areas the examiners are interested in. You will be asked to present your case summary, present and justify your differential diagnosis and, in the case of the Part II exam, go on to discuss possible management plans. To prepare for this:

- Know what is expected of you. Read the Royal College guidelines concerning the exam; these tell you about the content and structure of the exam
- Take opportunities to present cases (ward rounds, clinic, etc.)
- Practise presenting cases under exam conditions. For some of the mock cases, make sure that you are asked to interview the patient in front of the mock examiner. This is something that is rarely practised, but is important
- Seek supervised training in interviewing skills. Watch yourself presenting on video. This is a very effective way to identify what areas you need to change.

Mock clinical exams

In the Part I examination, candidates are told that the clinical case will be based on a case from one of the following, or a combination of these:

- General adult psychiatry
- Hospital liaison psychiatry
- Old age psychiatry
- Substance misuse.

In the Part II exam, no such specific guidance is provided. For both exams, make sure that you do mock clinical exams on each of the main areas of psychiatry. These are common problems seen in psychiatric practice, and hence are common in exams:

- Depressive disorder
- Schizophrenia
- Anxiety disorders
- Obsessive compulsive disorder
- Alcohol abuse/dependence
- Eating disorders.

If possible, do mock exams with a variety of **different examiners** who have different theoretical and clinical backgrounds. Do not just ask 'friendly' examiners who you know well. Seek out those

MOCK CLINICAL EXAM ASSESSMENT SHEET

Examiner: **Candidate:**

General: The ability to pick out the salient features of the case and present these clearly and coherently is stressed. The organisation of information is particularly important.

History taking: Is what is presented systematic and comprehensive with no omissions? Logically presented and structured?

Mental state examination: Systematic and comprehensive with no omissions?

Interview of the patient: Sensitive interview, good rapport, fluent interview style? Put patient at ease, good empathy? Good use of open then closed questions? Systematic and comprehensive with no omissions? The ability to firmly but politely control the interview without dominating, and at the same time cover the appropriate clinical questions quickly, clearly and efficiently should be assessed.

Physical assessment: Can recognise significant findings and identify their importance/relevance?

Overall impression/diagnosis of the case: Diagnostic skills, knowledge of aetiology including psychological aspects? Knowledge of diagnostic classification systems? Pay particular regard to social and psychological treatments, as well as purely physical approaches.

Presentation: Clear communicator and good delivery, articulate, clarity of presentation?

The assessment of **relevant physical factors** should be recognised in the mark. (7–10 minutes).

Interviewing the patient: Politeness and professional attitude? (5 minutes)

Overall mark: A general discussion with the candidate would probably be the most help rather than an overall statement of Pass or Fail.

Comments: Helpful ways to improve presentation and organisation of material?

(*Pass the MRCPsych*, Second Edition. Williams, Trigwell and Yeomans 2000)

with a range of examining styles. If there are any College examiners at the hospital where you work, you should try to carry out at least one exam with them as well. Be willing to accept their feedback and suggestions to change. Ultimately, however, you are seeking to develop a clinical interview and presentation style with which **you** are happy.

When you do the practice exams, try to obtain **specific** feedback. This will help you identify your relatively stronger and weaker areas. An assessment sheet such as the one above may aid this and can be used by others (e.g. your peers in a study group) to rate your performance. You can also use it yourself if you are analysing your presentation on videotape.

Predicting and practising cases

Try and remember that the hospital where you sit the examination will tend to have the same types of patients that you see in your own clinical practice. The hospital has to provide approximately 20–30 patients for the exams and these are therefore likely to include both inpatients and outpatients. Think through in advance how you will assess, present and manage each of the following clinical cases. It is not necessary to carry out mock exams on each of these, but you should think each case through thoroughly. You may find it useful to either write down full assessment and management plans of a 'typical' case, or to test and be tested by peers who are also taking the exam.

Write out full assessment and management plans for each of the following:

- Major affective disorders
- Schizophrenia (and drug-induced psychosis)
- Alcohol or substance abuse

- Anxiety disorders
- Obsessive-compulsive disorder
- Agoraphobia or other phobias
- Hypochondriasis and somatoform disorders

- Dementia (these patients will be accompanied by an informant)
- Eating disorders
- Any area that the examining hospital specialises in.

Do not attempt to visit or contact the clinical staff or wards of the hospital you will be examined at.
This can lead to you being disqualified from the exam.

It is possible that a patient with a learning disability or a child will take part in the exam. If so, they would always be accompanied by an informant.

Coming to the exam

Think:

- What impression do I want to give?
- What will I wear and how will I look?

How can I arrive on time?

It is surprising how often this causes problems. Expect the unexpected (traffic jams, rail strikes, losing your car keys, etc.). If you are late it will leave you feeling tense, pressured and unlikely to perform well. Consider staying overnight in a good hotel (not noisy). It is worth the money. A long drive with an early start on the day of the exam may be inadvisable, and being 'on-site' can make a big difference. If the hotel is poor or noisy, check out and move somewhere better. Passing the exam is worth more than the expense of an extra hotel bill.

Sometimes, particularly in Part II, patients may seem very complex. You can still pass by using a systematic approach to effective clinical assessment and presentation.

The clinical assessment

Engaging the patient

- Introduce yourself to the patient.
- Explain that you need to take some notes to help you remember (especially important if the patient is experiencing paranoid beliefs).
- Apologise in advance for having to interrupt them; say why (it is an exam; time pressures, etc.).
- Be polite and professional.

Be organised as you take the history

Nothing creates an impression of disorganisation more than a flurry of paper during the presentation. This can be reduced by a few simple techniques:

- Write on only one side of the paper
- Number the sheets
- Organise your information clearly as you take the history
- Use clear headings (Personal history, Family history, etc.)
- Consider writing the headings down at the start of the exam. This can help you pace your history taking, and also prevents you forgetting to ask about any central and important area.

It is not the place here to go through in detail how to take a psychiatric history. This is described in all basic psychiatric textbooks. A good description is in *The Oxford Textbook of Psychiatry*.[1] We suggest that you read the chapters on the psychiatric history and mental state in detail and repeatedly practise areas such as testing the cognitive state.

Presentation

While presenting the patient use a style most examiners will recognise. For example:

- Presenting complaint/ history of presenting complaint
- Personal history
- Premorbid personality
- Family history

- Social history
- Forensic history
- Past medical history
- Past psychiatric history (always including post-partum problems and deliberate self-harm)
- Drugs/allergies to drugs (do not forget depots or current ECT)
- Full mental state examination
- Physical examination.

Always mention the presence or absence of suicidal ideas and behaviour.

- **Maintain momentum**. You cannot afford to run out of time.
- **Leave gaps** between each area on your history sheets. You are likely to forget some questions and this allows you to fit in later information without creating an unreadable mass of extra notes scribbled in margins.
- You can always ask the patient what diagnosis they have been given, and also what treatments or investigations they have had. This can offer very useful clues.
- Aim to finish in 45 minutes. Ask the patient to stay while you review your notes and check what you have forgotten or need to clarify.
- Consider using a red pen or a highlighter to mark important key areas that you will later read out in the presentation.
- Thank the patient and mention that you will be asked to interview them again in front of the examiners.

An appropriate (often brief) physical examination should always be carried out and included in your presentation. This could include:

- Pulse
- Blood pressure
- Evidence of autonomic over-arousal (e.g. sweating, pallor, tremor)

- Stigmata of thyroid or liver disease
- Evidence of previous injury (self-cutting, etc.)
- Anything else that is clearly relevant (e.g. they use a wheelchair).

Clustering questions

A very important technique to learn is that of **clustering questions together**. In psychiatry, diagnoses are largely made by observing if particular symptoms aggregate together in patterns that are felt to represent specific disorders or syndromes. Most examiners have a model in their minds of the cluster of symptoms that make up each diagnosis (such as 'depressive disorder'). These clusters have been formalised in the various diagnostic systems such as ICD 10 and DSM IV. How then is this relevant to the exam situation?

Examiners do not have very much information about the patient you have seen. All they know is a basic written summary from the Senior House Officer looking after them. What you need to do is to **paint a picture** of the patient for them. In order to present this clearly to the examiners, it is vital to **cluster** symptoms together logically while taking the history, and therefore while presenting. This is the key to a good presentation. When, for example, you mention depressed mood the examiners will want to know if the patient fits their own (or the ICD) model of depression. They will therefore expect a description of not only how depressed the mood is, the presence of anhedonia, mood reactivity, etc., but also whether there is any evidence of 'biological' symptoms of depression, and to what extent the depression has affected the person's life.

Thus, if you are asking about depression **ask about all these areas at one time** so that your history contains a clear focused summary. Write the symptoms down on one part of the paper so that they are presented (clustered) clearly on your sheets, and hence when you present. Don't allow yourself to be distracted by the patient when taking the history. In some cases you may have to come back to clarify things later, but do this all on the same sheet of paper so that everything you have found out about a particular problem area is found together in that one spot. This will help you give a clear presentation.

Two typical 'clusters' of questions covering depression and anxiety are presented below. Each of these has a similar structure. Try to create your own individualised clusters which you will be able to remember easily. Practise these until you can go through them quickly and reliably.

Clustering symptoms of depression: a Five Areas Assessment

1. The situation, relationship and practical problems faced.
2. **Altered mood:** severity/ reactivity/ anhedonia, etc.
3. **Altered thoughts:** hopelessness, negative view of self/situation/future, suicidal ideas, etc.
4. **Altered physical/biological symptoms:** diurnal variation of mood, poor appetite, weight loss, etc.
5. **The altered behaviour/social impact of the symptoms:**
   - What have you stopped doing since becoming depressed?
   - What are you doing differently because of these problems?
   - How has it affected you, your family and work?

Clustering symptoms of anxiety: a Five Areas Assessment

1. The situation, relationship and practical problems faced.
2. **Altered mood:** How severe is the anxiety? Is it generalised or focused as a phobic state? Does the anxiety ever rise to a crescendo and cause panic attacks?
3. **Altered thoughts:** catastrophic thinking, jumping to the worst conclusion, worry, etc.
4. **Altered physical/biological symptoms:** Is there evidence of marked somatic anxiety? It can be helpful to cluster the questions by asking about evidence of sympathetic and/or parasympathetic symptoms, and also for any symptoms caused by hyperventilation:

Sympathetic nervous system:
- Rapid heart
- Palpitations
- Tremor
- Sweating
- Flushing.

Parasympathetic nervous system:
- Nausea
- Vomiting
- Loose motions/diarrhoea
- Frequency of urine.

Hyperventilation:
- Dizzy
- Blurred vision
- Depersonalisation/derealisation
- Sweating
- Dry mouth
- Chest pain
- Subjective shortness of breath.

5. **Altered behaviour/social impact of the symptoms:**
   - What have you stopped doing because of your problems (avoidance)?
   - What are you doing differently because of these problems (unhelpful behaviour)?
   - How has it affected you, your family and work?

Is there any evidence of **avoidance**? This has important implications for treatment.

Create your own **symptom-cluster checklists** asking about paranoid ideas/schizophrenia, alcoholism/substance misuse, eating disorders, obsessive-compulsive disorder, etc. You will find that the skills learned in doing this will also be useful for the time when you have to interview the patient in front of the examiners, because it will teach you to be organised, structured and clear.

What to do with the 'difficult' patient

Some patients may, because of their mental disorder, be difficult to interview. If this is the case:

- Take the history as well as you can
- Concentrate on completing as detailed a mental state examination as possible
- Try to control your nerves. The examiners will have been told by the exam co-ordinator of your difficulties. Tell the examiners what happened (once)
- What they want is your considered professional opinion based on the information (however limited) available to you. Try to adjust your mindset so that this is what you offer them
- Tell the examiners what you saw and heard, your current clinical opinion, what diagnoses could explain this presentation, your need for further information (state what you wish to learn, how you would seek this and your purpose in needing to know, etc.). You can still pass.

The vital quarter hour

Try to complete the basic history in approximately 45 minutes. In the remaining time check through your sheets while the patient is still in the room. There may be 5–10 minutes in addition before you go in to see the examiners after the patient is taken out of the room. This is an important time to gather your thoughts.

You do not have time to re-write or indeed read out the entire history for the examiners. Remember that the purpose of the history is to try to understand the person and their problems. You want to paint a picture for the examiners of the patient you have seen. Focus what you say in order to paint this picture effectively.

Structuring your presentation

Think in advance about the six areas you will be expected to cover:

1. Presentation of the history and mental state
2. Differential diagnosis (with justifications)
3. Aetiology – the three Ps:
   - Predisposing factors
   - Precipitating factors
   - Perpetuating factors
4. Investigations (social, psychological, physical)
5. Management (immediate and long-term; social, psychological, physical)
6. Prognosis (short-term, long-term).

Preparing to present the case

You have approximately 7–10 minutes to present the whole case. Of this, it is the opening few minutes that matter the most. It is during this time that you will present either a favourable or unfavourable impression. Examiners, being human, tend to label you as clearly passing or failing early on in the presentation. In our experience, it is quite difficult to switch between these labels once they are applied, therefore it is vital to have the 'right' label attached as soon as possible. How can you make this happen?

Prepare to pass

Prepare your opening few sentences. If the patient has been a difficult or poor historian say so now and possibly again later, but only once more. Do not overstate this. Next, **write out** the first two or three sentences of your presentation.

1. **A summary demographic statement**. Write this out in advance as one sentence only (see example below).
2. **The key problems** in the case. Write these out in advance as one or two sentences only (see example below).
   - What are the key problems?
   - You need to **focus** the history on these.
3. **Be ready to present the salient features of the whole history and mental state examination**.

Presenting the case

- State the **headings** whilst presenting the case in order to give clear signposts of where you are in the presentation ('Key features from the personal history include: . . .' etc.).
- Make sure that the flow of the history is **logical**, and present the history in a form that most examiners will recognise (see the discussion on taking the history above).
- Make sure that you communicate to the examiners that any important screening questions have been asked, even if there is no positive reply. For example 'On direct questioning there was no evidence of any of the first rank symptoms of schizophrenia', or 'There was evidence of early morning wakening, but no other biological symptoms of depression'.

Act of presentation

Remember:

- Keep calm
- Modify the following suggested model to fit your cases. If you already have an effective structure of presentation that you are happy with, then don't change it too much unless you want to
- Definitely do not change your regular style of presentation **on the day of the exam**. Get used to one style of presentation, and stick to it
- Make your presentation interesting; it helps to vary your voice tone as you present, and to make good eye contact with both examiners.

The following summarises the structure of a typical presentation:

1. **A demographic summary sentence.**
   'The gentleman I saw is Mr S. J., who is a 33-year-old married man who lives alone in his own house.'

2. **One or two sentences summarising the key problem areas.**
   This is the main focus of the history. **Write this out in advance.**
   'He has had problems which began after the ending of his

marriage four months ago. Since then he has been feeling **depressed, anxious** and **suicidal**. This led him to take an **overdose** that precipitated the admission to hospital. There are a number of associated difficulties including a lack of **social support** and isolation which have aggravated his situation.'

3. **Key parts of the rest of the history and mental state examination**. 'He presented two weeks ago with . . .'

   . . . then on to describe the main complaint (e.g. the depressive cluster of symptoms) and each of the other problem areas one by one.

   - Read these from your history sheets.
   - They should not need to be re-written.
   - Go through the rest of the history reading out the relevant items. Draw attention to positive findings, and important negatives (e.g. first rank symptoms example as before).
   - Use set phrases to save time: *'Mr S. J. describes a normal birth, development, childhood and schooling history. He left school at 16 and . . .'*. This informs the examiners that you have asked about these areas, but without spending valuable time stating this in full.

Presentation of the history should paint a picture of the person, their problems and the aetiological factors. Mention the relevant **p**redisposing, **p**recipitating or **p**erpetuating factors as you go through the history. After presenting the salient points of the history and the mental state examination, you will move on to present the differential diagnosis.

The differential diagnosis

Consider both psychiatric and physical differential diagnoses.

- There may be no single right answer.
- 'There are a number of possibilities which include . . .'
  e.g. '. . . a range of psychiatric and physical disorders can cause a similar presentation. In this particular case I would consider X, Y, and Z based on the following reasons . . .'.

- If it is obvious, however, state what you feel the diagnosis is.
- Show that you know that patients can change, and that your opinions are not fixed, but based upon the evidence that you find now at interview.

If it is very complicated, don't panic. Instead you can use a statement like: 'This is a very complicated case. After only an hour with the patient and without the chance to review the old notes or talk to an informant, I have a range of differential diagnoses, but at the present time I would not be able to put them into any definite order. However my differential diagnosis at present is . . .'

- If someone appears guarded, always consider including paranoid psychosis in the differential diagnosis.

State the diagnosis you favour at the present time. Using information from the history make the case **for** and **against** each of the differential diagnoses in turn.

Standardised differential diagnoses

You will be required to use the ICD 10 classification in the exams. You should therefore familiarise yourself with this classification. It can be very helpful to have pre-prepared a list of 'standardised' differential diagnoses for the common presenting problems that you come across. These are not lists merely to regurgitate, but instead help you to remember the range of diagnostic possibilities (both psychiatric and physical) for you to consider. Having these to fall back on can be a great help if anxiety levels are high and you are finding it difficult to think effectively during the exam. Do remember to only state these if you **really are considering them** for this particular case.

Only state actual possibilities. Don't just say 'or an organic cause of the disorder'. You must be specific about what you have in mind, and give evidence to support it, e.g. ' Hypothyroidism, in view of the history of loss of energy and marked weight gain'.

Again, only state these if you **really are** considering them in the differential for this particular case. Be prepared to justify your reasons for and against each of your differential diagnoses.

Differential diagnosis of depression using ICD 10

1. **Bipolar affective disorder**
   - Specify type of current episode
2. **Depressive episode**
   - Mild or moderate depressive episode +/– somatic symptoms
   - Severe depressive episode +/– psychotic symptoms
3. **Recurrent depressive disorder**
4. **Persistent mood disorders**
   - Dysthymia
   - Cyclothymia
5. **Adjustment disorder**
6. **Mixed affective episode**
7. **Personality disorder**
8. **Organic cause**
   - Hypothyroidism
   - Alcohol dependence
   - Other

Differential diagnosis of paranoid ideas using ICD10

1. Schizophrenia
2. Schizotypal disorder
3. Schizoaffective disorder
4. Persistent delusional disorder
5. Acute and transient psychotic disorders
6. Personality disorder (schizoid or paranoid)
7. Mania with psychotic symptoms
8. Bipolar affective disorder: manic or depressed +/– psychotic symptoms
9. Severe depressive episode with psychotic features
10. Recurrent depressive disorder: current episode severe with psychotic symptoms
11. Organic cause:
    - Drug-induced/alcohol
    - Temporal lobe epilepsy
    - Other (systemic lupus erythematosus, third ventricular tumour, etc.)

Investigations

Social

Do not neglect this area. It is a very important part of good psychiatric practice.

- 'I would obtain the old notes and read them.'
- 'I would speak to a relative, with the patient's consent.'
- 'I would speak to the ward staff and ask do they eat, sleep, mix, and laugh, etc.'
- 'I would consider other sources of information: GP, Consultant, etc.'
- Self-monitor: drinking or eating diary.
- Specialised reports can be requested if appropriate (e.g. social report).

Say **why** you would pursue each of these courses of action.

Psychological

Tests such as psychometric testing, mood rating scales, mood diaries, etc., may be indicated.

Physical

Think out in advance which investigations are **appropriate** for each illness. 'These could include . . .' (see box on page 90).

Use your common sense – say what you do in **practice**.

Management (Part II exam)

You need to show the examiner that you are competent, safe and sensible. It is important to say basic principles first even if they seem obvious:

- 'I would admit for a period of assessment' (if appropriate).
- 'I would want to treat each of their problems in turn . . .' etc.

- Bloods. State which and **why**. These could include full blood count (FBC), plasma viscosity (PV), renal, liver, calcium, sugar, vitamin B_{12}, folic acid, VDRL (venereal disease research laboratory) test and thyroid function tests (TFTs). Lithium levels may be appropriate. Know why these are performed, and the relevance if they reveal an abnormality.
- Urine drug analysis if appropriate.
- EEG if appropriate.
- Computerised tomography (CT) or NMR if appropriate.
- Blood alcohol levels if appropriate, etc.

Structured management plans

It is important to organise this part of the presentation in two ways:

1. Immediate and long-term management
2. Physical, psychological and social aspects.

As part of your exam preparation you should **write out typical structured management plans for the core psychiatric conditions**. Include affective disorders, schizophrenia, neuroses, substance misuse, eating disorders, etc. Although you will have to present a management plan tailored to the individual case that you see on the day, this will be easier if you have previously prepared typical examples in this way.

Prognosis

State your experience, not just papers. Consider:

1. The **classical prognosis** of this condition: make sure that you have learned the typical prognosis for common disorders (schizophrenia, depression, mania, panic, alcoholism, etc.).
2. **Specific features** of this patient which affect it in this case:
   - Previous history
   - Response to medication
   - Compliance with treatment
   - Social supports

- Characteristics and personality strengths of the patient
- Skills acquired
- Degree of intelligence and willingness to work collaboratively with you on their problems.

Key points

The exam involves:

- Meeting a patient for the first time and winning his/her confidence
- Obtaining a fully structured and relevant history
- The physical examination should be brief and concentrate especially on areas that will aid in establishing a diagnosis
- Planning your investigations and management according to your differential diagnosis
- Making sure that you come over as safe, sensible and professional.

REFERENCES

1. Gelder M, Gath D, Mayou R (1989) *The Oxford Textbook of Psychiatry,* Second Edition. Oxford Medical Publications: Oxford.

2. Williams C J (2000) *Overcoming Depression.* Butterworth Heinemann, Oxford.

Presenting to the examiners

Peter Trigwell and Christopher Williams

There will usually be two College examiners there when you present your long clinical case. Do not be worried if a third (the external examiner) is sitting in the background. He or she is present merely to record whether the performance of the examiners appears reliable and valid. He or she will make no contribution at all to your final mark, which is decided by the other two examiners alone.

Presentation techniques

- Passing the clinical involves presenting yourself well.
- Go in and act confidently.
- Do not say your name. State your **examination number** when asked (have it written down).
- Be polite and professional. Do not come over as too eager to please.
- Make eye contact with both examiners as you start presenting, **and** subsequently.
- If the examiners enquire about something that you have forgotten to ask the patient about, say that you would have normally enquired about this and why it would be important **in this case**.
- Don't shuffle the papers too much.

It is important to be adaptive and flexible. Carefully consider any suggestions the examiners make to you about diagnosis, etc. Do not reject any suggestions they make out of hand, but show that you can consider the relative evidence for and against a particular diagnostic possibility. The patient may have changed since the history was summarised for the examiners, or the patient may now be partially treated or have relapsed. Also, remember the clinical effects of medication or ECT on the mental state.

Difficult questions in the long case

Certain questions are often dreaded by candidates. This is unnecessary as they can be tackled in a straightforward and systematic way.

1. 'Present a psychodynamic formulation'

Sometimes an examiner will ask you to present a psychodynamic formulation of your case. Do not be thrown by this. You already have all the information that you require to answer this in your case history. Consider the person's:

a) **Mother and father** – their relationship with each parent; any evidence of excessive dependency or hostility, etc; any separation/individuation issues

b) **Personal history** – important issues/factors that stand out as being psychodynamically relevant, e.g. perceived abandonment or rejection; repeated patterns in relationships, etc.

c) **Defence mechanisms** – have any obvious defence mechanisms (e.g. projection, denial, etc.) been used in the past? Look for continuity of these defence mechanisms over time

d) **Features at interview** – any obvious defence mechanisms present during the interview; these may include avoiding painful issues, or crying when particular issues are touched upon; consider both conscious coping mechanisms and unconscious ego defence mechanisms; consider the patient's reaction to you (transference), and also your reactions to the patient (countertransference)

e) **Keep your formulation simple** – address it to the specific patient; say why these features are important, e.g. in considering treatment.

2. 'Describe this person's personality'

Again, this question is not as difficult as it may seem. You must comment upon three areas:

a) In your experience, is their personality normal or abnormal?
b) If it is abnormal, do they cause themselves or others to suffer? (i.e. do they have a personality disorder?)
c) If they do have a personality disorder, which one is it in ICD 10?

To do this well, you need to know the ICD 10 diagnostic criteria. If the patient's characteristics do not fully satisfy any of the criteria (as is often the case) say so:

'They do not exactly fulfil the criteria for any specific personality disorder. However they show aspects of certain ICD 10 personality disorders including. . . '.

3. 'Carry out a CBT formulation'

Adopt a five areas assessment approach:

a) **Situation, relationship or practical problems faced** – what situations cause symptoms? (e.g. going into a shop alone leads to panic); consider the social situation, their supports and practical problems faced
b) **Altered thinking** – how do they interpret what happens? (e.g. what are their fears during the panic attack?); identify any unhelpful negative automatic thoughts; identify possible core beliefs or unhelpful rules, e.g. 'I'm worthless/bad/unlovable . . .', 'Others let you down', etc.; identify any possible thinking errors (black or white thinking, jumping to conclusions, catastrophic thinking, mind-reading, etc.)
c) **Altered feelings** – anxiety; depression; anger, etc.
d) **Altered somatic/physiological changes** – biological symptoms in depression; arousal symptoms in anxiety/panic
e) **Altered behaviour/social impact** – e.g. stopping doing things in depression and withdrawal; reduced pleasure and sense of achievement as a result; avoidance and safety behaviours in anxiety.

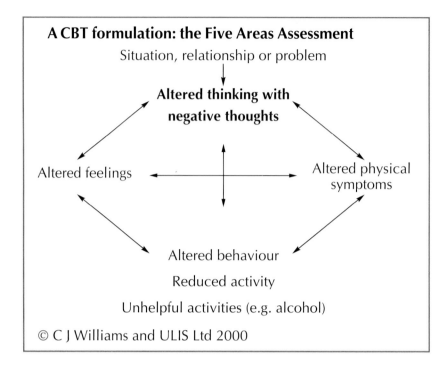

A CBT formulation: the Five Areas Assessment
Situation, relationship or problem
Altered thinking with
negative thoughts
Altered feelings
Altered physical symptoms
Altered behaviour
Reduced activity
Unhelpful activities (e.g. alcohol)
© C J Williams and ULIS Ltd 2000

Interviewing in front of the examiners

During the clinical examination in both Parts I and II of the exam, you will be required to interview the patient in front of the examiners for approximately 5–10 minutes. The purpose of this is to allow the examiners to gauge:

- Your professionalism
- Your manner with the patient (tact and empathy)
- Your clinical skills as a psychiatrist (listening skills, objectivity, interview skills)
- Your ability to elicit and demonstrate psychopathology (goal-directed, phrasing of questions etc.).

Many candidates find this a most stressful experience. It is rarely practised beforehand and, as a result, is a potential 'weak-spot'. Practise this part of the exam under examination conditions. It may be possible to do this within the setting of ward-rounds but it is better to do it as a separate exercise. You need to discover your potential weaknesses, and work to improve them. Ask yourself:

- 'Do I come over as a professional doctor with good clinical skills?'
- 'Do I show myself to be a warm, genuine listener, and at the same time can I take charge and direct the clinical interview?'
- 'Can I work efficiently to gather specific information in a clear way?'
- 'Which clinical symptoms do I find the most difficult to phrase questions about?'

The examiners want to know if you can control the interview, ask clinical questions competently and structure your time to complete the task in the time allocated, whilst being professional and polite to the patient. You must also come over as being genuine. If you have problems with being warm and empathic do not overcompensate. This will appear false. You are far better off in this circumstance if you adopt a professional manner that is polite but not brusque.

Typical questions the examiners may ask you with the patient present

There are certain questions which can be answered well in 5–10 minutes, and so are often asked:

1. Fact gathering
- 'Take a full alcohol history.'
- 'Assess the suicide risk.'

2. Eliciting symptoms
- 'Can you ask about their ideas concerning cleanliness and try to show whether this reflects an obsessional illness or not?'
- 'You mentioned that at times they feel threatened by those around them. Can you please ask a little more to try and decide whether these ideas are delusional?'

3. **Confirm or disconfirm a diagnosis**

- 'You mentioned earlier that it is possible the presentation may be caused by schizophrenia. Can you ask the patient more to try and examine this diagnosis in greater detail?'

4. **Specific task**

- 'Test the cognitive state of the patient.' (Or specified parts of this.) The Mini Mental State Examination[1] is a useful short test.
- 'Can you test the orientation and short/long-term memory of the patient please?'

Techniques

- Remember you have done this many times before.
- **Write down the questions the examiners wish you to cover**. If you are uncertain, ask for clarification.
- Set up the chairs that you and the patient will sit in so that they are at about 90 degrees and a comfortable distance apart reflecting your knowledge of good interview technique.
- Bring in the patient and introduce him or her to the examiners.
- Show the patient to their chair.
- Set the scene to the patient in front of the examiners. Show that you are aware that this is stressful for the patient as well. Try to help the patient relax and put them at ease. Say something like: '**Thank you** for coming in. It's **important** for me to be able to talk to you in front of the examiners for the purposes of this exam. Try to **relax** if you can, because it's me who is under the spotlight today, rather than you. I want to start by asking you **some questions which we've covered already**, but if you'll just bear with me it will only take **about 5 or 10 minutes**. Thank you. Well I'd like to start by asking you . . .'.
- Some examiners are irritated if you are too familiar with the patient. You should always refer to them as Mr, Miss, Ms or Mrs etc., and not address them by their first name unless they ask you to do so.
- Make sure that you cover all the questions that you are asked to.

- **Start from first principles**. Do not refer to things the patient has already told you during your first meeting with them. This can cause you to ask them very leading questions, and shows poor technique, e.g. 'I would like to ask you one or two further questions about the problems with checking that you mentioned earlier'.

- Make it obvious to the examiners which questions you are answering. If you feel that you are 'stuck' on an area, you can always move on and justify your decision later to the examiners. 'I have a number of things that the examiners want me to cover in only a few minutes, so we have to move on from this area.'

- **Try to ask open questions first, followed by more closed questions.**

- If the examiners have asked you to check whether a particular symptom is present do this quickly and efficiently. For example, if you are asked to elicit and see if a belief is a delusion (i.e. a fixed, false and unshakeable belief), then you must try and demonstrate that this is the case in the face of argument and evidence to the contrary, or that it is based on delusional evidence.

- **Decide on the ordering and prioritising of the questions**. For example, if you are asked to assess the long- and the short-term memory of the person, you should reverse the order of the questions so that you can give a test of short-term knowledge (e.g. 'I am going to tell you a short address . . .') at the **start** of the interview rather than at the end. This avoids an uncomfortable two minute wait at the end of the interview before you can test their recall of the address. As long as you ensure that you cover all the required areas, you can carry out the tasks in whatever order you think is best.

- Don't worry if the patient does not give the answer that you expect. Ask again in a different way. If at the end of a reasonable selection of questions things still seem unclear, move on. You can always be honest and tell the examiners if they ask you whether you felt you carried out an adequate assessment. If you feel you have not been able to confirm or refute the symptom, then you could for example say: 'I didn't feel that based on the replies that the patient gave there was evidence of thought disorder. I would want to spend more time with him/her to check this further'.

- At the end of the interview, thank the patient again and show them out of the room.

After the patient has left, the examiners may ask you what you noticed, and whether you were happy that you elicited the information adequately. Be objective in your reply. They may also ask whether any new information has been unearthed which may influence your differential diagnosis or management. If this is the case say so, again showing that you are able to take account of and integrate new information.

The present state examination

One of the worries that candidates often have is 'How should I ask appropriate questions?' Make sure you know how to ask about the presence of:

1. Psychotic symptoms:
   - Hallucinations
   - Delusions

2. Neurotic symptoms:
   - Depersonalisation/derealisation
   - Worry
   - Anxiety
   - Panic attacks
   - Obsessions/compulsions
   - Hypochondriasis.

Most people find that it is the 'psychotic' questions that are the hardest to phrase, as well as those asking about depersonalisation. Practise these in your everyday history-taking. If you are uncertain how to phrase the questions, look at questions used in the 'Present State Examination' (Wing et al[2]). These start with 'open' questions, have been widely used in clinical research settings, and have been found to be reliable. Many previous candidates have found these standardised questions very helpful.

Typical PSE questions include:

1. Delusional mood:
   - 'Have you ever had the feeling that something odd is going on that you can't explain?'
   - 'What is it like?'

2. Depersonalisation:
   - 'Have you felt recently as if the world is unreal, or only an imitation of reality, like a stage set?'
   - 'Have you felt that you yourself are not a real person, not really part of the living world, like an actor playing a part?'

3. Delusions of reference and persecution:
   - 'Have you felt that people are unduly interested in you, or that things are arranged so as to have a special meaning?'
   - 'Does anyone seem to be trying to harm you (trying to poison or kill you)?'

Key points
- **Write down** the areas you're asked to cover by the examiners.
- Be confident and take charge (arrange the chairs, etc.).
- Show the patient in and introduce him/her to the examiners.
- Show the patient to their seat and set the scene for him/her.
- If possible use PSE questions. Obtain a list of these before the exam and learn the most 'difficult' ones (e.g. depersonalisation).
- Elicit what was asked for. **Open** questioning is best, leading onto closed questioning.
- Impose your own structure and prioritise your asking of the questions as you think is best.
- Thank him/her again. Show him/her out and go with them. Be polite and courteous.

REFERENCES

1. Folstein MF, Folstein SE, McHugh PR (1975) Mini-mental state. A practical method for grading the cognitive state of patients for the clinician. *Journal of Psychiatric Research* 12 (3): 189–198.

2. Wing JK, Cooper JE, Sartorius N (1974) *Measurement and Classification of Psychiatric Symptoms.* Cambridge University Press: Cambridge.

Patient management problems (PMPs)

Christopher Williams

Patient management problems (PMPs) occur in the Part II examination only. They are set by a second pair of examiners, and will take place at the same centre and on the same day as the long case.

It is important to practice PMPs. Many candidates find them surprisingly difficult, simply because they have not become familiar with the technique. In reality, all you have to say is what you would do in best practice. You have been solving similar problems whilst 'on call' for the last few years. Be sensible and safe.

You will be expected to answer with a level of knowledge that is reasonable for someone of Specialist Registrar level. Do not be put off if the question is put to you by an examiner who you fear may be a specialist in the area of the question they ask. For example, if you have never done child psychiatry do not be perturbed by questions such as 'How would you treat urinary incontinence in a child by using the Star chart method?'. All that will be expected is for you to have a reasonable overall level of knowledge, and to understand the general principles involved.

PMP techniques

It is essential to be **systematic** and **organised** in your approach to answering PMPs. As the examiners ask you the question, try to identify the key issues/main problem areas. You may wish to jot these down on a piece of paper and make sure you address each of these during your answer. It is important, however, not to restrict your answers to only one area or aspect of the problem, thus going down a 'blind alley' and running out of things to say. Keep your answers broad. You need to have a clear:

- Opening
- Middle: impose a structure/keep it broad
- Ending: come to a clear end.

Opening

Try to avoid a lengthy pause. Your answer should have a clear opening. The following **three approaches** may help you start and structure your answer.

1. Key issues
What are the main issues raised by the question?

- Safety/risk issues.
- Issues of diagnosis.
- Management.
- Any Mental Health Act/Common Law issues?

'This question involves a number of different issues. These include the importance of being sure of the original diagnosis, the need for a full assessment, and also the difficulties of treating those with treatment resistant depression . . . '.

This has the advantage of showing the examiners that you can pick out the **key points/problem areas** quickly and have a firm grasp of the essentials of care. When you use this approach, make sure that you start off by describing the most relevant or important problem area first in order to avoid interruptions by impatient examiners.

2. Further information needed
Do you need any more information? Where from?

- To make the diagnosis.
- To decide on treatment.

- To assess the impact on the patient: what has he/she stopped doing because of the problem?
- To assess the impact on other people (e.g. carers, etc.).

'In this case I would wish to gather **further information** in order to clarify the diagnosis. I would talk to x,y,z in order to find out . . .'.

3. 'Talk yourself into the situation'

Imagine you have been asked to deal with this clinical problem whilst on call. What would you do in practice?

'If I was asked to go and see this case in casualty, I would begin thinking about how to manage the case on the way there. I would first go to the Medical Records Office, look up and obtain his old notes and quickly read them in order to find out more information. I would also phone the ward where he had been an inpatient and see if any of the nursing staff knew him . . .'.

Some people find this approach is most effective if you use visual imagery whilst talking about how you would deal with the situation. **This approach is often particularly helpful if you are feeling quite anxious.**

Do not begin to answer each question in exactly the same way. This may annoy and frustrate the examiners.

The middle/main component

Keep your thinking **broad**. Consider using different perspectives in your answer to aid this.

- Remember to consider **psychological** and **social** aspects of diagnosis and treatment as well as **physical** ones (e.g. effects on the patient, their family and work).
- What are the benefits and risks of treatment?
- Consider immediate and long-term treatment.

Remember that as you answer you are providing cues that will stimulate further questions from your examiners. Use this wisely. Try to avoid digging yourself into a hole.

Ending and possible problems

- Come to a clear end and look up, waiting for the next question/clarification.

Potential difficulties in answering PMPs

If you do not know part of an answer, say where you would go for appropriate and sensible advice. For example, if you do not know what drugs you can safely prescribe in pregnancy it is reasonable to say, 'I would contact Pharmacy and Drug Information and ask for further information.'

If the examiners appear to disagree with you strongly, be prepared to consider other possibilities. Feel able to discuss other diagnostic or treatment options. **Never get into an argument**, but if you think that you are correct, you should review with the examiners the reasons for and against each of the possibilities, and the reasons why you wish for the time being to stick to your first decision. Always show that if more information became available, or the person changed, you would be willing to reconsider.

The principles of effective answering of PMPs are illustrated by the following examples. Variants of these questions are commonly asked in the exam.

Example: treatment resistant depression

> 'A 65-year-old man has been weepy and depressed for three months. He has lost significant weight and there is marked anhedonia. He has been treated with Dothiepin for the last eight weeks and continues to be very low in mood. He has begun to express ideas of hopelessness and is feeling suicidal.'

The examiners may ask questions such as the following. These may be given consecutively to test the depth of your knowledge as you answer, or may be asked together all at once.

- How would you manage this patient?
- Would you make any change of medication? If so what would you do and why?
- You make all these changes and he continues to be unwell. How would you manage him now?

Spend about five minutes answering this question by jotting down your answers on a piece of paper. Try to be **organised** as you answer. What are the **main points** you need to cover?

- What are the main issues in this case?
- What further information might you need?

Possible components of the answer
Opening

1. Main issues, e.g.:
    - How to manage treatment resistant depression
    - Treatment issues in older patients
    - The need to clarify the diagnosis.

2. Further information needed, e.g.:
    - Is it a depressive disorder?
    - Is there a co-morbidity (physical or psychiatric)?
    - Compliance issues, etc.

3. Talk yourself into the situation: 'If I was seeing this patient for the first time in clinic . . .'.

Middle/main component of your answer

Expand on the areas mentioned in Opening 1 (main issues involved) or 2 (information needed).

Is the diagnosis correct?

In a 65-year-old man with weight loss, perhaps there is a hidden physical disorder (such as cancer). Has this been excluded?

'I would want to confirm that the diagnosis **actually is depression**. I would do both a full psychiatric history and also a detailed mental state examination. I would examine the person physically and send off appropriate screening bloods for physical disease. In particular, I would send off a full blood count to check for anaemia, and thyroid function tests to exclude thyroid disorder. If any other physical tests are warranted, I would request these (e.g. a chest X-ray in a smoker).

Check current and past management

- Ask other obvious questions: 'Is he actually taking the Dothiepin?'
- 'Is he taking an appropriate dose for an adequate time?'

'I would want to know if he was taking the tablets at an adequate dose. Within BNF guidelines, I would increase the dose as far as could be tolerated by the patient . . .'

Gather more information to make sure

State the information you require, how you would obtain it, and why you want to know:

'I would also obtain the old notes and read them. It would be helpful to talk to an informant, with the patient's permission. I would like to get a clear description from nursing staff, etc. of how the patient is during the day to see if his behaviour is consistent with a diagnosis of depression.'

One important focus of this question is 'How do you treat resistant depression?'. This is a classic and often repeated PMP. Make sure you have planned answers to such common management difficulties.

Do not neglect to mention **maintaining factors**. It is easy in a question such as this to only mention physical approaches to treatment. Abnormal personality, alcohol or substance misuse, and ongoing social and relationship problems are potential maintaining factors for depression. These would need to be addressed. Beware of hidden physical disease. The reactions of family members may also be relevant.

Ending

- Make it clear when you have finished your response.

The examiners may then either go on to another PMP, or add a further stem to the current question which will introduce a fresh angle to the problem. It is important to remember that there are a number of ways of answering any PMP. What matters most is that you are seen to be safe and sensible.

PMPs are usually genuine cases that have been encountered by the examiner setting the question. They represent real people and day to day clinical problems. As a result, practising PMPs with a local consultant or SpR can be helpful in preparing for the PMP exam. If you are confused by the question, be honest and say so. It is far better to clarify the question than to attempt it without understanding what is being asked.

Key points

Opening
- Have a clear opening using one of the three techniques outlined above ('main issues', 'further information needed', or 'talk yourself into the situation') and gain thinking time by concentrating on the key issues of the case.
- Don't use the same opening approach for each question.
- Be aware of the range of possible questions.

Middle
- Organise your answer clearly.
- Demonstrate that you are sensible and safe.
- Say what you would do in practice.
- Be divergent in your thinking and avoid going down a blind alley. Address each of the main problem areas.
- Use techniques to keep your answer **broad** and **organised**

(e.g. short- and long-term management; treatment benefits and risks; physical, psychological and social management options).

- Show that you are **flexible** and will consider the evidence for and against a range of diagnostic or treatment options if this is appropriate.
- Where appropriate, say that you would seek advice or information from others with more experience in that area.

Ending
- Come to a clear end.

Remember: Do not be dogmatic and where appropriate say that you would seek advice or information from others with more experience in that area.

If at first you don't succeed . . .

Kevin Appleton

Failing the exam

Not everyone passes the MRCPsych. Many people will have sat the exam one or more times previously. Failure will be experienced by a large number of candidates at some time whilst trying to pass both parts of the MRCPsych exam. I was such a person. This short section is dedicated to those people who may have a similar experience to me at some time. There are those who work long and hard, apparently covering all the topics thoroughly, but who still fail. This is a most disheartening experience and can cause a myriad of feelings including upset, and anger.

It is difficult to alleviate the sense of disappointment and exhaustion that follows the receipt of your application forms for the next attempt and condolences from the chief examiner. At this stage try to send off the form to **request feedback on your performance** as soon as possible. It is easy to be so fed up that you feel you never want to do the exam again. You may adopt an attitude somewhat akin to 'learned helplessness'. Failure will trigger off many thoughts that will convince you that Beck's Negative Cognitive Triad is an accurate model of depression. You are likely to feel pessimistic about yourself, the world and the future. You may begin to make negative predictions, and have the most catastrophic thoughts about the exam or your career. As with all such thoughts, they are both unhelpful and inaccurate.

Sending off for feedback can actually help challenge these beliefs. It can show you that **you are not bad at every part of the exam**. Realising this can be quite encouraging. You will have done better on some parts of the exam than others. This is useful information, because it shows you which areas of your performance you need to change.

Next is the difficult task of giving the bad news to others. Everyone wants to know if you passed but no one wants to ask you. Your colleagues may study you intensely from a distance to pick up clues (drooping shoulders, dishevelled appearance) before deciding whether to sit with you at lunch. Some people do genuinely wish to hear all about it and may allow you to off-load your sorrows. For others, try using a brief but positive sound bite.

At some stage you do need to accept the fact that failing an exam is a kind of bereavement. You need to give yourself time to recover before starting again. Try to be good to yourself, get plenty of sleep, and go out and do some of your favourite things. Do something different which is fun (and non-psychiatric). A short holiday away, or booking onto a course you have always wanted to do can be useful. There may also be practical matters that have been neglected during the intense revision and that need to be caught up with. Dealing with these will take your mind off the exam and put things in perspective. Family and friends may have had less of your time and attention recently, so take the opportunity to remedy this. They need to have you back for a while and you need their support and encouragement. Try to move your focus away from just the exam; in the long term failing the exam will not seem so important. No one in their right mind would choose to fail but if it happens it isn't the end of the world.

Looking to the future

You will have to try and work out exactly what did go wrong in your performance, and start to plan a strategy for another attempt. At a fairly early stage you should decide whether you are going to resit at the next opportunity or wait six months or more. This decision will have to be based on a number of factors. These may include practical matters such as house moves or any other foreseeable events that might make it just too difficult to give enough time to your revision. If possible, applying to resit soon is probably the best thing to do for two reasons. First, it helps you maintain momentum. Even if you take six or eight weeks off from learning after the last exam, your previous revision will be relatively fresh in your memory. You can use this as a firm foundation to build on. Secondly, there is only a short window of opportunity where you are allowed to apply for the exam. If you miss it, you will not be able to apply for the next sitting. If you are in doubt it is often best to apply and secure a place. For many people motivation to work comes back slowly with time, and this can be accelerated by having the focus (and financial commitment) of a booked exam. If you change your mind later, you can always choose to withdraw prior to the exam without this being counted as an attempt. There will be a financial penalty for doing this, however, as outlined in the College application forms.

The initial feedback from the College will tell you which part of the exam you have failed. The later feedback (which you have to request), may not arrive until a few weeks before the next exam. Do not wait until you receive this to go to see your clinical tutor, consultant, or other helpful persons who can help you at your next attempt. If you don't already belong to a study group this may also be the time to get together with three or four like-minded people who intend to take the exam at the next sitting. These groups can be a great source of support, encouragement, shared learning and knowledge.

After failing Part II, I felt that although I possessed a lot of theoretical and practical knowledge about psychiatry, I had not used or communicated this well in the exam itself. My second attempt involved a much greater emphasis on technique, after attending the Leeds MRCPsych Examination Technique course. Much useful work was also done in study group gatherings. This helped to focus my learning on exam-relevant information, and I would recommend it.

Appendix: Mind Maps®

Kevin Appleton

What are Mind Maps® and how can they help with the exam?

You will already be aware of your strengths and weaknesses when it comes to learning for exams. You will probably use techniques which you have (successfully) used over the years. Successful techniques allow you to structure, organise and integrate new information with the information that you already know in order to make learning meaningful. This is important because, particularly with the Part II exam, it is a practical impossibility to read through everything again in the few days before the exam. It is important to focus on key facts, so that these may be concentrated on in order to reduce the amount of reading you have to do when the work is revised.

Common and effective techniques to help you reduce the quantity of information you have to learn include writing short summary notes or using highlighter pens to focus in on key facts. Another, less common, approach is Mind Mapping®. This is not an approach that everyone will find intuitively appealing; however, some people find this approach to be a very helpful way of organising and learning information.

Mind Maps® are colourful, branching pictures or diagrams that can help your memory, thinking and organisation of ideas and information. They can make study more efficient by condensing more facts onto a single sheet so that very large amounts of information may be revised very quickly. In Mind Map® 1 (see page 116) the assessment and treatment of alcohol dependency is covered, together with the ways that alcohol problems can lead to presentation to the medical services. To maximise the effectiveness of Mind

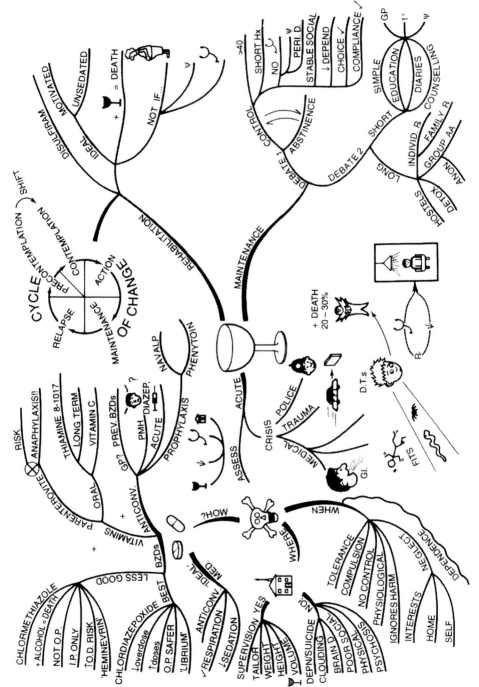

Mind Map®1. Alcohol – assessment, complications and treatment.

Maps® it is necessary to **produce your own** so that each sub-heading of the Mind Map® will trigger off associated pieces of information that are relevant to you. If you had Mind Map® 1 in mind during an essay, PMP or clinical viva, you would be able to answer most questions on this topic.

Mind Maps® work by increasing the cross connections and associations of stored information in memory. They use images or key words to anchor information and to trigger associations. It is possible to hold entire Mind Maps® in visual memory by this method and they are fun to use, making learning more enjoyable and revision less tedious. By using different modes of memory storage (e.g. factual, visual and colour), they increase the modalities and ways in which information can be remembered whereas linear text uses only one such modality.

How to create your own Mind Maps®

It is better to draw Mind Maps® across the horizontal axis of the page as the structure spreads out better this way. Start with a central image or icon. Recalling this from visual memory will trigger your recall of the whole map. Next arrange main headings or key words around this from the centre of the page. Sub-headings, lists and further details can then be added to each branch.

One heading or icon (e.g. head injury, as in Mind Map® 1) will come to represent, in your own mind, many other additional responses (sub-dural, penetrating, etc.). These act as anchors for surrounding text and help you to recall this additional information efficiently. Well organised information should result in an aesthetically pleasing map whereas poorly organised information will look a mess and will be less well recalled. To structure the content clearly on paper means that it must also be structured clearly in your mind so that drawing out the diagram is itself an effective means of revision. This is illustrated by Mind Map® 2, which itself summarises the use and production of Mind Maps®. You will see that the key elements of the linear text you are now reading are clearly and concisely summarised on one sheet of paper. This is both information-rich, and

Index